CHANGE YOUR MIND
CHANGE YOUR WEIGHT

CHANGE YOUR MIND
CHANGE YOUR WEIGHT

Dr. James McClernan
Psychologist

Foreword by
JEFFREY BLAND, Ph.D.

HEALTH PLUS PUBLISHERS
Phoenix, Arizona

CHANGE YOUR MIND
CHANGE YOUR WEIGHT

Copyright © 1985 by
James McClernan, Ed.D.

Library of Congress Cataloging-in-Publication Data

McClernan, James, 1935 —
    Change your mind, change your weight

    Bibliography: p.
    Includes index.
    1. Reducing — Psychological aspects. 2.   Mind and body. 3. Obesity. I. Title [DNLM: 1. Diet, Reducing — psychology. 2. Obesity — psychology — popular works. WD 212 M478c]
RM222.2.M433   1986   613.2'5'019   85-24890
ISBN 0-932090-15-X

Illustrations by Len Boro

Typography by CLS Typesetting

Published by
HEALTH PLUS PUBLISHERS
P.O. Box 22001, Phoenix, AZ 85028

Printed in the United States of America

Dedication

*To my mom, Ethel, and sisters, Lois and Kay,
for teaching me to persist, laugh, and care.*

ACKNOWLEDGMENTS

Change Your Mind/Change Your Weight *reflects the efforts and contributions of:*

Mary Mirocha for her caring support, editing, and creative thoughts;

Dr. Jeff Bland, for writing the Foreword and for his biochemistry and nutritional input;

Drs. Scott Rigden and George Leonard for their kind words;

The helpful staff of Shape Magazine, *Judie Lowellen, Robin Crosby, and Pat Ryan;*

Karen Jensen, Karen Lyman, and the staff of Health Plus Publishers for their extra efforts to give this work a touch of panache;

Schick's Shadel Hospital and Drs. James Smith and Fred Lemere for the opportunity to do my research with their support;

John C. Lincoln Hospital and the staff at Cowden Center for their help with my on-going programs;

All the kind and sharing members of my weight-loss programs over the years for the many kindnesses and insights they have given me.

FOREWORD

Dr. Jim McClernan's new book, *Change Your Mind/ Change Your Weight,* takes a no-nonsense approach toward one of today's most complex and common problems — eating disorders and weight management.

The problem is that most commonly used diets and weight-loss programs have very poor success rates because they do not deal effectively with the base causes of excess weight or with the cultural and psychological aspects of weight management. Losing weight, in itself, is not a problem. The real questions are how to lose weight (fat) in the right manner while maintaining muscle, and how to lose in such a way that you have long-term effectiveness in your weight loss.

This, to a great extent, has to do with changing the psychosocial experience of eating and the psychology of foods in our culture as well as individual behavior patterns. Dr. McClernan has dealt realistically and thoroughly with these concepts from the basis of his experience and research as a psychologist and a professional working in the wellness movement. His book deals very effectively with the multifactorial aspects of maintaining proper body composition and addresses such topics as stress, exercise, motivation, procrastination, hidden fears of becoming thin, and lifestyle, as well as simple eating habits.

It's too easy for us to look for simple answers to complex problems, and *Change Your Mind/Change Your Weight* puts the problem of weight management into the appropriate social millieu which deals with cultural values and normative structures of our society. Everything from food production to food distribution, the economics and politics of eating, and the past experiences of an individual, including his ethnobiology, all play a role in establishing who might be likely to have excess body weight versus who will not. Dr.

McClernan addresses all these aspects of food and eating, and helps provide a clear understanding of their impact on weight management.

This book is a fine tool for use in implementing a holistic approach to weight and health management that is individualized for the reader's specific needs. I am convinced that *Change Your Mind/Change Your Weight* will make a vital contribution not only to the achievement and maintenance of proper body weight, but also to a general sense of wellness and health improvement.

Jeffrey Bland, Ph.D.
Linus Pauling Institute of
Science and Medicine

PREFACE

Only ten percent of those people who solicit aid from commercial programs or weight-loss diets are successful for any more than short periods of time.

This is the woeful statistical assessment of the magic illusions promoted by the national fat industry. Ninety percent of the anguished help seekers end up disillusioned, angry, poorer, psychologically depressed, and feeling weaker, hopeless, and helpless, possibly in a weakened state of health. One recent study has indicated that sixty to seventy percent of those who attempt to lose weight through their own efforts are successful at losing the weight and maintaining their weight loss five or ten years later. The conclusion that may be drawn is that most people who seek assistance not only want magical cures that allow them to lose weight without effort, but they may even perversely resist or work *against* weight loss. *Change Your Mind/Change Your Weight* is a facilitative tool which will provide you with information and guidance that is insurance against being "ripped off" by the fat industry, and show you ways to avoid sabotaging your own efforts.

Exercise is extremely important. Although this book is not filled with pictures of pretty people in a variety of exercise positions, it clarifies and defines safe exercise and the many options and places available for it. More importantly, it explores how to change attitudes about exercise so that it becomes a regular, life-long, preferred activity. Dr. McClernan looks at procrastination and provides information on how to stimulate motivation from within so you won't have to rely on a Jane Fonda or a Richard Simmons to provide the impetus to keep fit.

The book approaches nutrition in the same manner. Instead of advocating a particular weight-loss diet and filling the book with menus and recipes, Dr. McClernan is more concerned with teaching you to prefer a natural, healthy diet that is right for *you* and to become aware of what your body needs as it goes through its continuum of changes. The book emphasizes the development of a *preference* for healthful food — to avoid getting into that *struggle to resist* certain "forbidden" foods. Learn to spontaneously make good food choices instead of relying on a highly structured weight-loss diet, counting calories, and reading food exchange tables.

Exercise and nutrition are only two of the basic factors involved in losing weight. This book considers the **WHOLE PERSON:** body, mind, beliefs, and support systems. It explores emotions — the subconscious reasons why people want to stay overweight or fear becoming thin. It relates being overweight to stress, careers, education, and relationships. In other words, it deals with the reasons why so many people do not have long-term success with weight-loss diets, drugs, gurus, starch blockers, protein supplements, gimmicks, wraps, plastic suits, staples in the ear, etc., etc. Also, the book examines why some things that might otherwise be useful, such as hypnosis, accupressure, aerobic dancing, and organizations such as *Weight Watchers, TOPS,* and *Overeaters Anonymous,* are not cures in and of themselves. Unlike dangerous and radical medical procedures such as intestinal bypass, stomach stapling, stomach wraps, balloons in the stomach, or wiring the jaw shut, which are unnecessary, unhealthy, and counterproductive to a quality life, this book promotes health, self-confidence, and the ability to determine your own goals.

During the early seventies, Dr. McClernan conducted a broad research experiment for the Schick Company at their Shadel Hospital in Seattle, Washington. It was at this time that he determined there is no single cause and no single cure for obesity. Each person is different and functions as a whole unit with all aspects of the self interacting with the environment and its cultures. Weight problems are seldom simple. There is much more involved than taking in more calories than are burned.

People with serious weight problems are seldom understood or appreciated. It is difficult to see them as ordinary people with ordinary thoughts and emotions. Often they are the brunt of jokes and the victims of prejudice, and their sensitivities and pain go unnoticed. You can benefit from reading this book no matter what your weight concern might be. You can help someone else with a weight problem, correct or prevent your own weight problem, or you can simply grow as a person.

The philosophy and theme of this book are simple and clear: **You can change.** You can learn to take charge of your life. You can feel fulfilled instead of just full. You can be aware of yourself, be at peace with yourself, and you can develop coping skills and potentials to maintain this high quality of life. Whether you use the book's meditation techniques, family relationship arrangements, or one of the aids found in the Appendix, the main thought to hold on to is that *you are in charge* now and always, if you want to be. Your freedom is there for you.

Change Your Mind/Change Your Weight provides you with guidance in setting up your own program, which you will personalize to fit your circumstances and needs. Most of all, the book will help you in identifying and letting down psychological defenses and building up confidence to take charge of your own body.

Although some factors such as specific organic conditions, which Dr. McClernan discusses, may inhibit weight loss, there will be few people who will need additional help to achieve their desired goals.

TABLE OF CONTENTS

cont. next page

INTRODUCTION

Dear Reader:

This book is intended to be used as an opportunity for you to take a non-judgemental, non-critical, non-threatening look at yourself and your life. A chance to look at the whole you — body, mind, and beliefs. A chance to become aware that you can learn to take charge of not only your weight, but also your life. A chance to accept the responsibility for yourself and the **FREEDOM** that goes with it. A chance to release yourself forever from dependence on external magic to solve your problems, including overweight. This book can help you get where you want to go — be who you want to be. It can point the way for you to realize your fullest potential as a human being.

Through my many years of experience as an educator and counselor, in hospitals and universities, I have, I think, gained a great deal of insight into the things that motivate people to lose weight or to stay fat. I'd like to share some of this experience with you. I'll be telling you about some people I've worked with, and perhaps you'll identify a little of yourself and your concerns in someone else's story.

The main thing I want you to keep in mind as you read this book is that YOU are the key to your own success. I believe that this book can be of help to you in setting up a holistic program to help you lose weight and gain a healthy, fulfilled lifestyle, but **you** will be the person who can take the credit for any success you have in solving your weight problem. The book is simply a facilitative tool for you to use.

If you're looking for a magic pill or a magic diet, this is not the book for you. If you're ready to explore the idea that the answer to being overweight lies beyond counting calories, depriving yourself of everything you like to eat, and forcing yourself to sweat through some kind of exercise you hate, then read on.

Where's the magic? **THE MAGIC IS IN YOU!**

James McClernan, Ed.D.

SPECIAL NOTES

*DEFINITION OF TERMS USED FREQUENTLY
THROUGHOUT THE BOOK:*

Holistic — the synthesis by each person of their bio-physical, psycho-emotional, and transpersonal-spiritual self into a harmonious whole.

Existentialism — the belief that humans are responsible for their actions and who they are; that they are free to choose what they want to become within their physical and intellectual limitations. A never-ending process through life, with change and choice as its root.

Humanism — the idea that each person has value and to promote the welfare of that value gives greater worth to all humans; also that we are more than just cause and effect. We use emotion and intellect to motivate and choose.

Self-actualization — the active physical/mental quest to seek out the unending human potentials to be more than we are in all aspects of ourselves, as well as the higher values by which we may live.

No information presented in this book is intended to be, nor should it be interpreted to be, diagnostic or prescriptive. Before beginning any exercise, diet or supplementation program, it would be wise to consult a holistically-oriented physician and consider carefully his advice.

1

FOOD AND THE HUMAN CONDITION

FOOD IS NECESSARY FOR SURVIVAL

Food and life are inseparable. Every cell in our bodies requires nourishment; without food our strength, energy, and resistance to disease rapidly diminish. Without food we die.

Obtaining, storing, and distributing food and all the related materials, products, and services requires that a great many people spend a great deal of time making it possible for us to eat. For all social units, as well as for individuals, food is a focal point. Nations, states, cities, neighborhoods, the family, animals — all living things require nourishment on a regular basis, and we either compete or cooperate for our share if we are to go on living.

Food has not always been, and is not always now, easily available. The ways and means we have had to secure and share food have not been adequate to our development as a species. Because of this, food is not only involved with our physical, environmental, social, cultural, and governmental existence, but also our emotional existence. As thinking animals, it is amazing how illogically we have always related to each other and our mutual sustenance of life.

Although our technology for providing more than adequate amounts of healthful, tasty food has developed tremendously during the course of human history, we still have not learned to live with nature, each other, or ourselves where food is concerned. Most of us are dependent on others for our food. We tend to be fearful that we will get too little food, too much food, or the wrong food. We become greedy or overly-generous; over-involved or under-involved. We become disconnected from our nutritional needs and rely on quantity and taste to guide our choices. We tend to respond as much or more to our emotional needs for food as to our dietary needs. Our self-image, acceptance of one another, status, health, and love have all become interrelated with food.

In countries such as ours where food is in abundance, there are still some people starving while others are overfed and undernourished. As large corporations are rapidly taking over the production of food, fewer and fewer of us are able to grow food for ourselves. We have become more highly educated, yet we are just starting to learn what we should eat, how it affects us, how to prepare it, store it, and serve it. If we do have a basic understanding of nutrition, we seldom are aware of when our needs as an individual change or how to adjust to these changing needs. It is amazing that we can be so dependent on any one thing (food), be so involved with it in all aspects of our lives, and yet have so little knowledge of it. The information and the means to acquire it is there, and the need to understand food and our relationship to it becomes ever greater. I urge you to bear with me while I point out the extent of our involvement with food, and maybe you can begin to see how we have come to be so confused and emotionally blind to food and the human condition.

TOTAL INVOLVEMENT WITH FOOD

From the beginning of man's time on Earth, food has been involved in every aspect of our being. Until we are assured of an ample supply of food, it is exceedingly difficult to progress in our social, spiritual, or sexual lives.

The first occupations were hunting and harvesting food. Food has always been a medium of exchange, and bartering is still used extensively in various parts of the world. Agribusiness has become a huge and powerful industry. Wars have been fought over the control of rich agricultural lands. The ability to control food represents *POWER*, be it the strongest cave man eating his fill before those physically weaker get their share, or modern government subsidies to the farmer, food stamps, foreign aid to Third-World countries, feeding huge armies, or trade embargoes against the USSR. **Whoever is in control of the food has the power.**

Religions have always been very much involved with food, from sacraments of bread and wine, to live sacrifice of animals and even human beings to appease angry gods; from the Last Supper, to allowing cows to roam untouched in India while millions starve nearby; from rain and harvest prayers and dances, to radical diets and fasting. Many modern religions still maintain doctrines concerning food. The ways in which religion has influenced our concepts of food and consumption are many and varied.

Through **reward and punishment,** food has been used to condition and train us. I was manipulated with food as a child by parents who had the best of intentions. If I was a "good" boy, I would get a treat (sweets). If I was bad, there was a cold supper, or no supper. If they wanted me out of sight for a time, I was sent to the store for ice cream, candy, or pop. Schools and prisons use food as manipulative tools, as do governments, in controlling whole populations. In communist countries, hero awards, medals, and better living conditions go to those who produce more food for the cause. When we play a hard round of golf, we reward ourselves with an extra beer. If we've made it through a family trauma, we deserve a dinner at the best restaurant in town, and on and on it goes.

Food is often the primary focus of a **celebration.** Thanksgiving, Christmas, birthdays, vacations, and other special occasions often mean we have permission to gorge ourselves. When we think of entertaining, whether it be picnics and beach parties or dinner theaters and dancing, it usually includes eating fattening foods. To impress family and friends, we often serve special food we've prepared ourselves. Food can thus be associated with love, caring, and even self-esteem. Mothers may believe they are loved primarily because of the foods they prepare. Some cooks view food preparation as an art form from which comes great self-esteem.

Our relationship to food deepens as we view our **social status** and food. Where we eat, what we eat, and who fixes it can all become symbols of who and what we are. Different classes of people prefer different types and qualities of food. The quality of food is very much a factor in poverty, in that people who are poor tend to have poor diets, producing weaker children whose mental capacities and physical energies are reduced. It is a short jump from good food to good health and vice-versa. People with better diets tend to live longer and are sick less often, as well as being brighter and stronger. Where we were once inclined to view plump people as healthy and prosperous, we are now more inclined to view slim people in this way.

Food once had, and is beginning again to have, importance as **medicine.** Our first medicines were herbs and food concoctions. Now we are going far beyond mother's chicken soup to total lifestyle changes that often include vitamin supplements and individualized diets for better health. Educating people about the quality of food and its effect on body and mind has just begun. Athletes and holistic health educators, biochemists, nutritionists, as well as churches, governments, and some medical people are promoting this education as a life-long process in our overprocessed and polluted world. How we assimilate and burn food energy as individuals is a continuous need we are just now starting to examine. By studying certain groups of people around the world who have extended their lives beyond their eighties and even into their hundreds, we know that diet not only influences the way we age, but also how long we live.

Some foods are also used as **cosmetics** to promote beauty. Nothing is more attractive to me than a healthy person, and if this person has had the beauty of health very long, it is obvious that a healthy diet is involved. The beauty that goes beyond just being some "socially approved" degree of slim, to being present in the eyes, skin, hair, and all organs, comes with a healthy diet.

It is easy to go from beauty to **sex,** as the two are certainly related. Food is involved in the sexual appetite because food involves our senses. These senses strongly influence our feelings, and the same senses are heightened by sexual activity. Food itself is sensuous. We even have diets that are built around sexual activity — oral needs transfer from food to sex, which in a liberated age is not uncommon. We use sexy people to sell food in ads, and the association is made again.

Finally, if our world should fall apart due to war or economic disaster, those who are able to feed themselves have a better chance of survival. Even if a person simply wants to escape the mad, high-pressure conditions of today's society, the accessibility of food must be a primary consideration. Be it a person or a nation, the ability to feed oneself can virtually mean **independence and freedom.**

Briefly, I simply wanted to point out in this first chapter that we, as human beings, are totally and completely involved with food from the time of feeding at our mother's breast the first day of our lives, to our last meal. It reaches every corner of our lives, affects our attitudes, values, lifestyles, motivations, and fears, as well as our weight and health. ***To understand this in the beginning is a basic necessity to the rest of what you will read in this book.*** Our awareness of what food means to us has been growing by leaps and bounds since the space age began. Even doctors and scientists are beginning to acknowledge its importance to all aspects of our lives.

APPEARANCE COUNTS IN THE GAME OF SUCCESS

Unfortunate as it may be, research indicates that generally, when success is measured in terms of money, position, fame, and power, we learn that we must compete and do better than the next person to be "successful." We also learn, in a society that values the rewards of success, that physical attractiveness is a significant part of what is needed to win out over the next person. Our identity as people has to do with our self-confidence in adjusting to life. If we feel good about ourselves, our chance for success improves. If we then succeed in some way, our confidence grows. If, as a teenager you made the team or were popular with other students, you are less apt to be overweight. If you graduated from college, own a house, and drive a nice car, you are still less apt to be overweight. If you have been acknowledged as being physically attractive, you are least apt to be overweight. My follow-up studies of graduates from a state university clearly indicate no connection between grades in college and success, as measured by income and position. Students with a "C" average overall did as well as "B" and "A" students. *Personality* and *appearance* factors weighed much more heavily.

Richard Nixon, in his first run for president, was said to have been defeated (at least in part) because he could not compete with the more handsome and youthful John Kennedy in their appearances on national television.

Psychology Today magazine ran an article a few years back called "Beauty and the Best," which pointed out that attractive people are initially viewed as brighter, more honest, more personable, healthier (physically and mentally), stronger, etc. Success seems to come more easily and rapidly to attractive people, and a big part of being attractive in our society at this time is being *thin!*

If you are one of those fortunate people who achieves success (even moderate success), you then have the means to live a more hedonistic (pleasure-seeking) lifestyle. You don't have to worry about the cost of food; you are required to do less physical work; more people wait on you; you often have expense accounts, longer and more frequent holidays. It seems that success gives you a much greater opportunity to get fat and soft. However, statistics show that rich people, as a group, are a good deal thinner than people at the bottom of the economic scale. Certainly we have all seen celebrities on talk shows speak of their many efforts to stay thin. They tell of fat farms, special crash diets, and fasting. On the whole, celebrities are a thinner, better-exercised group than the average population because they need to maintain their physical attractiveness to hold on to the positions they have.

At the other end of the economic scale, poor people often have extra pounds, in part, because of the type of food they eat. They often have a very high sugar and fat content in their daily diet. They tend to buy food products that will fill them up and stretch their food dollar: more refined carbohydrates, sugary foods, and fattier meats; and less fresh fruits, vegetables, and lean meats. Then too, when a person is poor, the taste of sweet food can be one of the few sweet things in life. In addition, poorer people are generally less well educated and often not as aware of the quality of food or its effect on their health.

Sixty percent of the middle class is estimated to be overweight. They are striving to achieve success, are in a hurry, and eat handy fast foods, frozen dinners, and over-processed foods loaded with sugar, salt, chemicals, and empty calories. Often, for this group entertainment means eating out. *It is easy in this society to be overfed and under-nourished.*

THE SCENE IS CHANGING

A growing interest in prevention and developmental health has been coming about in the last ten or fifteen years. Health food stores, spas, racket ball clubs, etc., have mush-roomed. Whole grain breads and natural everything (including beer) have come from the back-to-nature movement of the sixties when young people were searching for a simpler lifestyle. It is "in" to jog and read labels. This movement seems to be led by the young people from upper-middle income families.

We are an affluent society that has been striving for opulence and hedonism, but it seems that those who have achieved this status are now choosing a simpler, healthier lifestyle; a lifestyle that fits in with the new ecology move-ment. Those who are concerned about ecology won't harbor fat or polluted foods in their bodies. Hopefully, this interest in the quality of life and self-responsibility for personal health will come to be the prominent and dominant theme in our society. It is the best way I know to reduce the cost of health care. What each of us does as an individual will determine what happens to the family, the schools, the churches, the communities, and ultimately the world.

2

CIRCLES OF FAT – THE MANY CAUSES OF OBESITY

It does little good to cite statistics such as those indicating that Americans have increased their food intake by six percent since 1976. The question still remains — WHY? We have more knowledge of fat's detrimental effects on health, both physical and mental; we have more medicine and technology to deal with it; a great many more professions are concerning themselves with finding answers and treating and facilitating those persons plagued by weight problems. *Why* are so many people continuing to gain so much?

ROOT CAUSES OF FAT

In my opinion — and research findings bear this out — there is no single cause, as there is no single cure, for weight problems. There are major categories of root causes. It appears that the interaction of several factors contribute to obesity. The following is a list of what I generally consider to be main root causes. I will simply list the root causes, with the exception of organic conditions, which we will discuss in some detail.

* Personality factors
* Heredity
* Environmental conditioning
* Living circumstances
* Emotions
* Physical addiction
* Sedentary lifestyle
* Basic motives (power-achievement plus affiliation)

ORGANIC CONDITIONS

Some organic difficulties caused by heredity factors or breakdowns in body regulators, as well as certain glandular disease, can cause some people to have a more difficult time burning calories than others. Although scientific studies are being done, the following possible factors are not hard-fact proof, and even if they were, no known cures or treatments to change the underlying causes are available at the time of this writing, so it should not preclude the overweight person's efforts to avail himself of the suggested methods of weight loss known to be safe and reliable.

Excess fat cells. Excess fat cells, a greater than average number of fat cells in a given part or all of the body, are a result of overfeeding in infancy and leave the victim permanently prone to taking on added weight.

Low basal metabolic rate (BMR). The BMR is the amount of energy expended while at rest. Some obese people burn approximately twenty percent less energy at rest than do people of normal weight, thus they require twenty percent less food. Fat tissue is metabolically more inert than lean tissue. The BMR decreases when less food is eaten, and when less energy is used, more fat stays in place.

Low body temperature. Obese people usually have lower body temperatures. Calories that would normally go into heat production are stored. This lowered body temperature increases the appetite, causing the obese person to eat more, thus compounding the problem.

Less brown fat. Obese people may have less brown fat than lean people, or what they do have does not burn properly because of a faulty trigger mechanism. Brown fat is a source of heat found around various internal organs. It *may* function as a minifurnace, burning excess calories. It *may* also have to do with the temperature of the hypothalamus, which signals desire for food when it is cool.

Hypothalamus damage. The hypothalamus, located at the base of the brain, is where the appestat (eating control center) is located. When this tiny regulator is damaged, it may cause overeating.

Cholecystokinin (CCK). CCK is a chemical produced in the brain and intestinal tract. It is believed that CCK calls a halt to eating. When the hypothalamus is damaged, it cuts off this chemical. CCK influences only the quantity of food eaten, not the way fat is deposited.

Adenosine Triphosphatase (ATP-ase). ATP-ase is a biochemical enzyme which may be found in all tissue cells of the body. It acts as a pump to push appropriate amounts of sodium and potassium in and out of the body's cells, consuming calories and generating heat in the process. A slowed pump may cool the hypothalamus, which stimulates the appetite until it gets warm enough. Low levels of ATP-ase may cause brown fat to burn less well. Most obese people are expected to have lower levels of ATP-ase than lean people. The rate of energy use *may* be controlled by ATP-ase.

Insulin. The hormone insulin regulates the amount of sugar burned in the tissues. A consequence of obesity is hyper-insulinemia. Overproduction of this hormone promotes the storage of calories as fat by speeding both the entry of sugar into the fat cells and its conversion into fat — "fat begets fat." Theoretically, it may be that an increased level of insulin in the brain chemical called the cerebrospinal fluid could help notify the body that it is too fat. The problem would then be how to get an increased level of insulin only in the cerebrospinal fluid.

Many sub-categories exist under each root cause, and all circumstances need to be considered. To say that caloric intake exceeds caloric expenditure is only a description of behavior, not a cause.

DETERMINING THE CAUSE OF OBESITY

It is possible that one obese person could have developed a larger percentage of fat tissue than the average person by growing up in a family of big eaters who belonged to the "clean plate club," and had the economic means to eat as much as often as they liked. This same individual's cultural environment may hold traditional beliefs that "chubby" people are healthy, happy, and more attractive. It is also possible that this person could have an injury to the ventro-medial region (satiety center) of the hypothalamus, plus, he* may have developed Cushing's syndrome (excess cortisol). Along with these multiple causes for being obese, it is then possible that this same person could develop a self-image or psychological problem which could also contribute to additional obesity. To add to the complexity of the situation, when this person begins to be grossly obese, he would become more sedentary, burn up fewer calories, and become even more efficient in the storage of calories.

You can see that trying to determine a single contributing cause for *one* person's fat would be impossible after the fact. Trying to determine a single cause for the *general population* of obese persons is truly impossible. Just attempting to unwind the psychological factors by themselves is extremely difficult.

A combination of factors is almost always responsible for obesity. Even though the factors seem to be all environ-

---

* When I make references to "him," "his," or "he," throughout the book, I do not intend to refer exclusively to the masculine gender. This is simply a means of avoiding the awkwardness which results from the constant use of he/she, his/her, etc.

mental, psychological, or organic, it is unlikely that there is one single cause, but rather a combination of environmental factors, or a combination of psychological or organic factors. Therefore, no single cure is going to meet the needs of any one person, let alone *all* obese persons. A comprehensive approach would seem necessary, with adjustments unique to each individual, based on determined needs.

POOR SELF-IMAGE
CONTRIBUTES TO OBESITY

Often a weight problem, or the inability to deal effectually with it, seems to be due to a poor self-image, which encourages self-doubt and feelings of inability to make decisions with commitment. Failure to make decisions increases loss of self-confidence, which leads to feelings of anxiety and depression, which in turn leads to poor self-insight, ineffective behavior, and failure. Failure, of course, returns us to poor self-image. It is at this point that you look for comfort, often found in inadequate or self-defeating adjustment mechanisms such as food (dependence in the form of sensual comfort). Because the adjustment mechanism is self-defeating, the whole cycle of events becomes more intense; you increase your efforts at inadequate adjustment (eating), and the condition grows worse. Becoming fat is, of course, seen as proof of failure, and adds to the poor self-image, which in turn becomes harder to change.

The influence of rapid changes and uncertainties in our society (marriage, divorce, family life, sexual mores, religious ethics, uncontrolled economics, unemployment, war, crime, elimination of the individual, etc.) puts additional pressure on you, and you may feel you have fewer places to turn for support, reassurance, success, and security. You will, perhaps, begin to feel more alone in your efforts to change your cycles. A feeling of helplessness and apathy can set in and you slip further and further into a loss of direction in your life. You may become disconnected from your feelings and awareness of yourself and the way you interact with the world. Confusing thoughts are repeated: "What's driving me to eat?" "Why can't I control myself?" It is common, then, to become more rigid in your ways, because your habits represent security (eating for comfort, and fear of failure in change). Some people may become chameleons and match the color of their present circumstances (dependence on, or direction from whomever or whatever is handy). In either case, it can take a traumatic happening or a long painful process of individual search and discovery with the help of others before change will take place.

> **Magic cures seem inviting because magic would be expedient and easy; but, alas, where *is* the magic? I believe that it is in each of us. The question is, how to bring it out? The answer may not be clear or easy, but certainly is worth finding.**

Where "hard core" dieters are concerned, dieting is not the answer, nor is exercise, alone. Even if you have organic injury or hereditary physiological problems, weight loss is still possible. If environmental conditioning has encouraged inappropriate eating habits and/or lack of exercise, you still have the ability to change, even though that change may be hard.

FAT CAN BE AN EMOTIONAL GIRDLE

Fat can be used as a problem upon which to focus, whereby you avoid facing deeper, more frightening concerns. Also, when you derive sensuous comfort from eating, it seems to temporarily calm you, and you forget about your inner emotional pain. For example, a housewife who has been at home raising children for several years finds her family needs a second income, but she has become paranoid about her work skills. What a convenient handicap fat becomes! She thinks, "nobody will hire a fat person like me; I must lose these extra pounds before I try to find a job." Somehow, the fat never comes off. This woman is perhaps correct in believing that fat people have less chance in the job market, but the point is that she has a means (the fat) of avoiding going out to retest her long-unused job skills. Of course, no effort — no failure.

Does what you are reading make you nervous or angry? Is the idea of fat as a crutch hitting too close to home? Listen to your body. It will tell you where your fears are. If you don't deal with them, the emotional girdle will get tighter and the pain will last longer.

If you have all the knowledge and resources and remain overweight because you don't use them, the chances are good that your feelings are acting as an emotional girdle. It can be frightening to examine your emotions. Looking at your fears is especially hard when you think the fears may be justified — that you *really are* a bad or weak person.

When you leave your emotions unexamined for long periods of time, it's easy to become afraid of them and to find elaborate means to avoid dealing with them — such as a girdle of fat. When you, on your own initiative, bring your fears to your conscious attention, even the worst fears quickly dissolve. Wearing a girdle of fat to keep the emotions contained is painful, and the more emotional data it holds in, the more painful it becomes. It is time to examine all the things that may be going wrong in your life now. To deal with each concern you have, one at a time, will remove a great deal of pressure from your girdle, and you will need less fat to hold the emotions in.

OBESITY IS AN EMOTIONAL GIRDLE WHEN:
. . . you know what good diet is
. . . you know what good exercise is
. . . you have the support of others
. . . you know plenty of gimmicks
. . . you know how your environment affects you
. . . you know if heredity or organic injury influence you
AND YOU ARE STILL FAT.

Finding your emotional buttons (fears) takes time and effort, and it means being open, honest, and objective with yourself and other special people in your life. After you find the emotional buttons, you still need to deal with each concern in a manner that won't overwhelm you. This may mean seeking help — sometimes professional help. Most of the time you can deal with most of your concerns if you approach them on your own initiative. Go slowly; stop when the pressure gets too great, but don't retreat. Simply keep the fear up front and (mentally) hold your ground until you feel comfortable there, then move forward slowly again. If the concern seems too great, you may have to work it out and get comfortable with it in your head first. We will review this technique in more detail in a later chapter.

Of the many ways change can come about, **realizing that you are free to change** is the best, because it has the built-in assurance of being self-directed. This builds confidence, leads to longevity of change and strength to seek additional self-improving change — to break the self-defeating cycle. The psychodynamics of perpetuating obesity can be extremely complicated and involved. The starting place and motivation for change can be different for each person. Breaking the circles of fat is difficult at the start, but gets easier as the self-actualizing circle grows. Because the change is hard to make, success offers a real chance to like yourself.

Your body, your mind, and your belief systems are in continuous interaction. Each part of you affects all the other

THE WHOLE PERSON

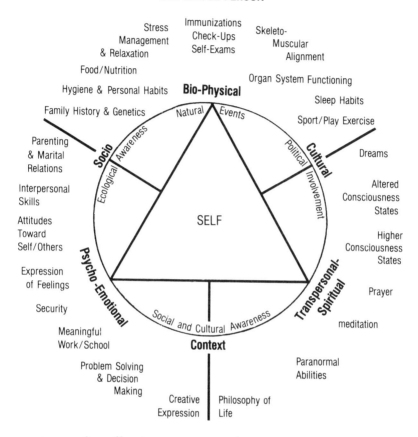

parts, so the effective way you relate to your world is as a single unit. Thus, starting a cycle into obesity, or away from it, is a simultaneous relationship, not an isolated occurrence. Begin to think of yourself as a whole person, and realize that all of the things that you do that are either self-defeating or self-improving will influence the direction of your circle. The answers you require are all within you. Chapter 18, along with the rest of this book, will help you put it all together. As your self-awareness, action, and self-confidence grow, so will your speed of change to a new, happier, thinner, healthier life ahead.

3
WOMEN AND FAT

Unlike their male counterparts, overweight women usually not only readily acknowledge their condition, but also often go to extremes to achieve thinness. Conditions such as *anorexia nervosa*, in which the sufferer experiences chronic fear of appetite for food due to underlying emotional factors, and *bulimia*, where bingers use vomiting or laxatives to get rid of what they have eaten, are almost exclusively female phenomena. Millions of women spend their entire lives in pursuit of an elusive thinness that they may find difficult to even imagine in their own minds.

> **The message is clear: females are told in one way or another from the time they are children, that if they are overweight, they aren't going to be loved, they aren't going to achieve in their careers, they can't be attractive, and they aren't really feminine.**

Women are the targets of advertisements for magic weight-loss cures. Have you ever seen a Hollywood movie where the fat girl gets the leading man? In recent years there have been a few TV series where the leading character has been an overweight female, but her size is often the brunt of jokes.

Most clothing manufacturers do not make their best and most attractive line in sizes for larger women. Their models are thin and willowy, and the clothes they make look best on thin and willowy women. Businesses that offer positions dealing with the public will commonly not hire women who are overweight, whereas with men, it is mostly in the upper echelons of the business world that weight becomes an obstacle to career growth. A few years ago, a female cheerleader in a mid-western high school was kicked off the cheerleading squad because she was five pounds overweight. Although I can certainly think of exceptions, in terms of success they *are* the exceptions rather than the rule; and for those women who have achieved, it has often been in spite of their weight — or sometimes even because of it — which is to say, maybe if a woman's other options for happiness are somehow being denied, it could be that she puts a more complete and exclusive effort into her career. Regardless of whether or not this possibility exists, in a world that places a premium on slimness, the overweight woman is probably forced to work harder to achieve the same ends as her thinner competitor.

Mothers, peers, doctors, businesses, and the media are all sending the same message to girls and women of all ages — *you've got to be thin to be valued and acceptable.* Under this kind of pressure, how can women avoid feeling an obsessive-compulsive concern with their size? They become willing to pay a tremendous price to get thin and stay that way. Women have also been given contradictory messages as to how to achieve slimness. Until fairly recently, women were taught that almost any physical exercise, other than dancing, was not feminine. This was especially true if a woman was *good* at a particular physical activity. Being physically active was for males, while sedentary activities were thought of as more appropriate for women. Even though the feminist movement of the last couple of decades has brought a dramatic change in the attitudes and behavior of a great many women, the large percentage of them still feel that femininity and perspiration are not compatible.

With women's magazines such as *Shape, Fit, Self, Slimmer,* and *New Woman;* media talk shows; spas; the military; women's professional/collegiate sports; the medical world; and movie stars now broadcasting the news that the well-conditioned woman is "in," the pressure has increased more than ever to be trim.

Another part of this whole sociological transition is the mixed messages regarding the emotional role of overweight women. When I worked as an instructor and counselor at a state technical university where males outnumbered females three-and-a-half to one, the ratio of students that sought counseling was seven females for every three males. This is just one of the many statistics which indicate that not only are females more open to counseling, but also that they feel a stronger need for, and are more desirous of help in attending to personal problems.

When first requesting counseling, the students were asked if they preferred a female or male counselor. Over fifty percent of the female students indicated they preferred a male counselor, implying that they perceived males as being better able than females to help them deal with their personal problems. Although I'm sure the same survey done with today's college women would yield an improved result, the fact remains that women have been conditioned to believe that they are inadequate and need help in attending to personal problems much more often than males, resulting in more inaction and passive "waiting to be saved" — not only from the world, but also from themselves. Until a woman no longer seeks external magic to save her and realizes that the way in which she buys into the male/female role blocks her chances of refocusing internally on her own strengths, her chances for meaningful changes in her attitudes about herself and her ability to take action against the unwanted pounds are limited.

In addition to the mixed social, emotional, and physical stereotype conditioning a woman is subjected to, there are other attending contemporary, economic, and family inhibitors that make her task of weight loss harder than that of males.

The wife who has an outside career may have less time and energy to devote to exercise, relaxtion, and eating properly, depending on how liberated her husband is. The single mother definitely has to be more organized and dedicated to accomplish all that she has to get done, and usually she must do it on a lower income than a male. The lower income not only gives her fewer opportunities (i.e., babysitters, maids) to find time to add healthful activities to her lifestyle, but also increases her stress, and then her emotional eating urges may increase as well. For example, it is still most common in divorce that the woman ends up with the full care of the children. If she wishes to have a regular exercise routine, when will she be able to accomplish it? In order to feed the kids, get them off to school, and work in a half-hour or hour of exercise, it may mean that she has to get up at 4:30 A.M. to make it to work on time. If she exercises after work, she has a conflict with shopping, other errands, getting home to be with the kids and to clean house and prepare dinner. Exercising after dinner may mean interference with evening activities she's involved in, running alone in the dark, getting a babysitter, etc., etc.

Loneliness, a big contributing cause of emotional eating, is also harder for women to counteract for several reasons. Because beauty/slimness has been made such a premium for women, once those extra pounds are there, the female tends to be more self-conscious about going out to the spa, the beach, or any social occasion. She tends to feel more inadequate and avoids crowds or takes a timid, "I'm not worthy/attractive" position with male prospects. Not going out as much as men, only going to certain places, or having to avoid certain activities, she is not apt to meet as many prospective partners as a single male might. Again, being a single parent makes the whole dating situation even more difficult and her feelings of not being worthy still greater.

Women are becoming more assertive in establishing relationships with men, but a woman who is overweight, and therefore feeling inadequate and unattractive, is apt to feel very reluctant to be assertive in attempting to initiate relationships with men. Males have always been taught to, or have been approved of, for being aggressive with women, and if they have no children to take care of, have a higher income, and less social emphasis to be attractive, they are much less likely to be timid or to stay at home and feel unworthy than are their female counterparts.

> *All of this is not to say that women cannot deal with the circumstances they face,* or even to suggest that their weight concerns are not dealt with as well as a man's. It is simply to acknowledge that while men and women have some concerns in common, there are some very real differences. Paying attention to the differences offers more options in dealing with them.

I will not cover in this chapter the steps to overcome these concerns and problems, since they are presented in other parts of the book. But I will point out again the need to acknowledge and use humanistic-existential behavioral and holistic principles in dealing with the special concerns women have.

4
MEN AND FAT

From my own experience and observation, it appears that overweight males have some distinct differences from overweight females. Probably the clearest difference is the man's reluctance to openly seek help for overcoming obesity. While women often believe they can't solve their problems without some kind of outside help, men get hung up in the opposite way, believing that they should *never* need help, and resenting or putting down counseling assistance.

In attempting to gather male subjects for my obesity research at Shadel Hospital in Seattle, Washington, it was necessary to go to great lengths to secure even a minimum number of participants. By using special incentives and obtaining help from their families and physicians, I was finally able to convince eleven men to start the experimental weight-loss program. At the same time I was struggling to get even a few males into the program, it was necessary to turn away over one-hundred female volunteers, many of whom were angry because they weren't accepted.

Why? Why do these situations exist? Are more women than men overweight? Do women have a harder time dealing with weight than men? Don't men care about being fat as much as women do? What are the answers? Although it is difficult to find much hard data on the subject, there are a few possibilities to consider.

Among "normal" people, women do have a higher percentage of body fat than men — approximately ten percent more. The number of men above their "normal" size is also less than that of women. However, it is true that men are dying faster and earlier than women of fat-related illnesses. Also, society does value and reward slim people more than fat people — both men and women — so why don't men involve themselves in weight-loss groups as often as women?

It is likely that many factors can influence the male's reluctance and female's eagerness to seek help for obesity: the fat industry and its promotions, female dominance of existing programs, cultural training, ego needs, education, occupation, and family and ethnic traditions are a few of the factors.

If you, as a man, drop into a meeting of almost any obesity program, you are likely to find you are one of a very few — or possibly the *only* male in the room. Even with the proliferation of "unisex" businesses, a great many men are not yet totally comfortable in any predominantly female setting such as the beauty parlor. Joining *Weight Watchers, TOPS,* or any predominantly female group is apt to be uncomfortable for most men. In my own experience of being the only male in an otherwise all-female group, I find that I tend to seek the background so I don't stand out as much in the group. When I'm in charge of a totally female group, I feel a little more anxiety, since I know mine is not a female view of the world. Men are apt to be intimidated by female conversation and embarrassed, perhaps, in the way a voyeur might feel if he should be caught peeping. If the leaders of the predominantly female group are also female, the uncomfortable feelings for the male in attendance are multiplied. To a man in this setting, it looks like a "woman's problem," and he is there to seek help from females for *his* female problem. In fact, just the idea that the male sees himself as seeking help *at all* from *anybody* flies in the face of macho conditioning. The feelings are ones of weakness and failure — more as a male than as a person with a weight problem.

Until recent years, the message for most males has been that they should be stronger, wiser, more independent, and the leader and protector of females, especially where physical matters and emotions are concerned. One way that an overweight man might view his obesity is that it represents weakness. Unlike an accident or a germ, fat is something the man feels that he should be responsible for, or in charge of. Because fat is something hard to hide, his male ego is constantly damaged, and he feels vulnerable. In his mind, he can't be Robin Hood, only Friar Tuck — considered to be a good guy, but comedy relief — the guy who never gets the girl.

Since the common view of obesity is negative, some men take an alternative view which at least a small minority of people appreciate. This view is that bigness equals maleness and strength. It allows some fat men to see themselves as admired by woman and feared by men because of their size and strength. The more of anything a man has than another man can be rationalized to be good because it buys into our competitive society which gives us all the urge to outdo the next guy. When you see a man with a large beer belly pat his stomach, laugh, and roar out, "It's all paid for!" he may, at that moment, actually feel proud of his obesity. If a man chooses to view his obesity as positive, why get rid of it? To the best of my knowledge, women do not have this option. The only positive view of femininity of which I am aware is to have height in proper balance with weight. To be considered pretty, a woman must be trim, and preferably not too big in bone structure. Small, frail, and weak have always been synonymous with feminine. This view seems to have changed some, but not to the point where fat can be looked at positively.

The fat man who wants to see his large size as being more masculine may simply be attempting to cover his own fears of weakness. He may feel that if he tried to change, he would fail, or without the uniqueness of his size he would lose his standing in his social group. Men see other men as unforgiving, and especially unforgiving of physical weakness or fear in other men.

Because of my many years of college and work as a psychologist, you may think my awareness and training would have freed me from these negative, macho, chauvinistic feelings, and it probably has helped; but the primary identity with the old male stereotype dies hard. I did find in my own research that the male white-collar workers with post-high school education were not only better able to handle the ratio of males to females in a weight-loss group, but also they were more appreciative of the psychological and philosophical parts of the program. Males with higher socio-economic levels were more tolerant and appreciative of weight programs dominated by females. The longer the lower-income, less-educated, blue-collar worker would stay in the group, however, the more appreciative he would become of the whole program. The macho, laboring man tended to see life more simplistically and himself as being more rugged than his more educated, higher-income brother. Thus, asking for help of any kind was less apt to be approved of. Men appear to be as vain as women, if not more so, but the vanity may take different forms.

I found that a change of attitude was influenced more in group encounters. Men started to see the women as equals in most ways and felt more accepted as men if they acknowledged their own problem with obesity. For some of these men, it was the first time they had ever expressed their feelings of fear and anxiety to any woman, and a strong bond of friendship, rather than sexual challenge, was created. Certainly this is one of those points where fat becomes the catalyst for greater personal growth.

Even though gains were made with male-female relationships, the men were clearly more competitive with the women than with the other men, although they were competitive with the men in the group also. The men felt that they had to be more aggressive with their exercise and diet and take off weight faster than the females. They were more aggressive in the small groups as well, whenever it was felt to be a challenge. "I can be more open with my feelings and show less emotion than you," was what they seemed to say. If the challenge wasn't clearly a challenge, the men would be more closed.

> **I challenge each man who reads this to design his own program and use some of that macho chauvinism to develop a holistic mode of life that will bring out all his hidden potentials, including that of living as long as females.**

In a classroom situation, men asked fewer questions and made many more recommendations than the women. Men came in for counseling only when it was a scheduled part of the program, while women requested private sessions frequently. Aversion conditioning (faradic shock, a painful but non-damaging electric current directed across the skin, put together with the eating of certain favorite fattening foods to create an aversion to the food) was a part of the research project at Shadel Hospital, and it was noted that there seemed to be little or no difference that could be attributed to gender when it came to tolerance levels for pain. This part of the program was done in private, which may account for the lack of difference.

In conclusion, I want to suggest that at least for men, sex role identity seems to have a significant influence on how, or even *if*, they deal with obesity. Males may be more inhibited about their feelings or about openly seeking help, but their need to establish a healthy body and lifestyle is as great as for women.

What I want all of you — both men and women — to realize is that *you* can take full credit for all the progress made in your program: your decisions, feelings, and actions will be your own. The challenges are many, and much more than just "fat."

One man in the program said to me, "You don't see a three-hundred-pound man on *every* street!" For him to relinquish his extra one-hundred-fifty pounds was a major threat to his identity, his social role in his community of friends and associates. How would he stand out in the crowd? To this man, his fears seemed real and well-founded. He didn't realize the wonderful potentials that would emerge through his holistic weight-loss program. Gradually, he began to realize that he had worth as a person. People liked him for who and what he was becoming, not just because he was bigger than everybody else. He established a new and better relationship with his wife as well as his friends and colleagues. His work began to improve. People praised him for overcoming his weight problem, and soon he was more of an admired celebrity than the odd person in the crowd. Most of all, I doubt that he ever felt more like a man.

5
THE FAT RIPOFF – WHERE'S THE MAGIC?

What I have to say in this chapter may be offensive or embarrassing, because you may be, or may have been, a part of what I call the "fat ripoff." You might think I am speaking unfairly or inaccurately, judging from your own experiences. Please keep in mind that I am speaking in general, and products and programs should be judged by you as an individual. And, if you accept the responsibility for becoming aware, you'll have the choice of making use of what is good and appropriate and discarding the rest. I'd also like to preface what I am about to say by acknowledging that from the best sources I can obtain, as well as my own research and observation, only a small percentage of those overweight people who try any given technique or gimmick will succeed in getting extra weight off and keeping it off for a prolonged period of time. Dr. Albert Stunkard, in "Don't Sell Habit Breakers Short," *Psychology Today,* August, 1982, determined in his overview summary that only about ten percent of the people who seek assistance with weight reduction have long term success (five-ten years later), while sixty to seventy percent who attempt to lose weight through their own efforts experience long-term success. When a person is committed to the goal of losing weight, the means chosen become more or less important in terms of success. When a person is determined, he will succeed. The means is important, however, in terms of general health.

Fat reduction, like alcohol and tobacco sales, is a very big business in the United States today, and big business has needs of its own. Many people look to obesity for their livelihood. When there are a lot of people making a lot of money from weight-loss products and services, ending the national weight problem becomes difficult and complicated, indeed. And, as we will see in later chapters, often the very people with the extra pounds are the ones who want the problem to continue.

Hundreds, perhaps thousands, of products and services of every kind and description are being offered to the over-eater. One major company offers a large array of highly fattening, nutritionless, sugar-laden foods, while at the same time making millions of dollars from the sale of specially packaged diet foods and conducting "fat" club meetings around the United States.

GIMMICKS REPRESENT MAGIC

Gimmicks in the fat industry take many forms, but they all represent a little magic — something that is supposed to take weight off easily. By themselves, gimmicks are ineffective; however, if you take a holistic, self-aware, self-responsible approach to weight loss, you may be able to select one or more gimmicks and use them to your own advantage without being ripped off. (See the Appendix for a list of usable gimmicks.)

The focus of gimmicks is strictly on *fat*. Thus, gimmicks mislead and create false hopes. The user avoids dealing with all the other factors contributing to his condition, and of course, is disappointed and upset when he realizes that the gimmick isn't working. Gimmicks often are ideas advanced in books — so be careful of *all* books.

If you wish to incorporate a gimmick into your holistic program, ask yourself the following questions:

1. Is it vastly overpriced for the materials or services you get?
2. Could you devise something similar on your own?

3. Are you trying to avoid your own responsibility?
4. Could it create a dependency?
5. Does it have the potential to be physically or emotionally harmful to you in any way?
6. From your past record, are you apt to make good and regular use of it?
7. Do the people who are offering it know what they are doing? What is their track record? What are their credentials?
8. Are these same people getting rich from it?
9. Do these people seem to care about you as a complete and whole person?
10. Is it offered as a magic cure?

An example of a doubtfully useful gimmick is the cellulite fighter kit, coming to you complete with soap, lotion, and special washcloth to wipe fat off the back of your legs. (Sounds like a good deal?) Another example of a useless fat reducer which has sold by the thousands is the sauna garment which melts fat from you while you sleep. No exercise, no diet, just sleep while wearing the magic plastic garment. It is hard to tell how many people are too embarrassed to admit they have tried gimmicks like these. The worst of all these "magic" methods are the over-the-counter and prescription diet tablets sold in untold millions. Even if you lose some water (therefore, weight), you do not change your lifestyle or gain a better self-image, and you could be subjecting yourself to the risk of harmful side effects.

Drugs and hormone shots also deceive and disappoint you if you're looking for a "magic cure." Usually with gimmicks, you have little or no weight loss, and the expensive gimmick is quickly abandoned. With drugs and hormone shots, you go to a doctor's office, receive some attention, and as long as you continue this program, the weight loss continues. You may even attain your ideal weight. However, as soon as medication is discontinued, the pounds usually begin to return. Most of the time more weight is regained than was lost in the first place. Such failure damages your confidence. Future attempts will be more difficult to start, and you will be more apt to *believe* you will fail, which will result in a weak effort. In the process of using the drugs or hormones, real biological damage may have been done, you will have spent a great deal of money, and most importantly, you will have learned little or nothing — except that **there is no magic out there.**

"FAT" CLUBS, CLASSES, and GROUPS

Many "fat" clubs and groups have sprung up around the country. Some are large national organizations — business ventures run for profit where, directly or indirectly, you can spend a great deal of money. Some are nonprofit and low cost, some local or regional, some are run by health spas, hospitals, or large businesses for their employees.

As part of a total comprehensive individualized program, clubs and groups can be effective. However, most groups are neither holistic or individualistic, or even humanistic. Many groups are supportive to some extent, but may use embarrassment and pressure techniques, which negate whatever support they intended to provide. Most groups give little or no individual attention. Usually one program or plan has been designed for all. Often the group member becomes dependent on the program instead of learning to become independent.

Clubs and groups usually emphasize only one aspect of what should be a holistic program. Diet or exercise is the usual focus, and they touch lightly or not at all upon other aspects of a total program. Individual psychological counseling and spiritual aspects are most commonly left out. Because these groups are designed to perpetuate themselves, you, as an individual, become secondary to the life and size of the group.

Many clubs and groups do not have complete or adequate facilities to conduct a holistic program, and even more commonly do not employ trained professionals. Thus, you often get inadequate and incomplete information. At best, you may find personnel with a high level of enthusiasm and energy, but without the skills and knowledge to deal with individual needs.

Many organizations keep no comprehensive records and have little or no follow-up on members once they have been out of the group for one or more years. Fantastic claims, often based upon very weak research, are used as promotional data for the program — promoting the illusion of magic. All of this, however, is not to say that a group that is right for you can't be extremely helpful. I'll talk more about support groups in Chapter 18.

The benefits you receive from a group are a sense of belonging and a feeling that other people close to you understand what it is like to struggle with fat day after day. A good group will also lead you to assert your individuality, let you know you are safe within the group from social judgements or rejection, and that you can expect support, as well as positive confrontation as you share with other members. You should feel a sense of responsibility to the other members of the group to treat them similarly, and to learn from the interaction.

Groups, like gimmicks and drugs, however, can be a means of escape from self-responsibility. They can be a socially comfortable group with which to identify. I've known many overweight people who confessed to going to fat clubs just to get out of the house or to have a group of overweight friends to go out for lunch with after meetings. One group *advocates* being fat and protests public preference for being thin. It serves as a sanctuary for fat people. A place for them to feel sorry for themselves, to give up, to complain about how abused and misunderstood they are, and to rationalize their condition. This might just as well be a suicide club!

When people use a group as a means of losing weight, the big hope may be that someone or something will save them from themselves, or that fat will suddenly be thought of as socially acceptable. They are looking for magic.

Groups for overweight people are often superficial. Members are commonly reluctant to confront one another or to be confronted. Supportiveness among group members is extremely important, much more so than criticalness. When sincere caring confrontation (not criticism) is joined with strong group support, it is a combination hard to beat. These two elements aid in bringing about a high level of trust in the group, and trust, in turn, enables more positive confrontation and support. Superficial groups keep their focus on external subjects (i.e., food). Topics are not personalized, shared, or explored as to origins or meanings. Confrontation in a strong, well functioning group isn't used to attack or accuse, rather it is sincere meaningful questions and the sharing of emotional reactions to one another, leading to greater self-awareness. Support from a well developed group doesn't mean only listening, protecting, and comforting. It also means modeling, being open, giving feedback, and facing the hard challenges together.

Programs that are primarily formal classes with a one-way flow of information from the teacher/therapist, bring about little change in you. Experiential learning and emotional sharing within a strong group are much more effective in the long term. Experiencing and sharing require action and involvement which make it difficult to remain a spectator and avoid changes or self-awareness.

Your readiness to enter in-depth groups can be noted by the way you respond during the initial orientation interview. For example, when clients are seeking magic to save them, they listen selectively. Words that are hard to hear are screened out. When I say to you, the prospective client, "You won't be told what to do; rather you will be given options with which to initiate your own program activities," you may then respond with an eager smile and nodding head, asking, "Which parts of the program will I have to do first and how long will it take to reach my goal?" The idea that you are in charge may be so foreign or undesirable that you won't wish to hear it at all. It is easy to see how vulnerable someone in this state of mind is to being ripped off by the commercial fat industry. Often times, even the well-intentioned weight-loss provider is as blind as the client. Both the provider and the client have an emotional and/or financial investment in the interaction, and both want to have their needs met. Both parties may be ready to settle for a few quick pounds of water-weight being lost, with no meaningful awareness of the underlying problems or no permanent change accomplished.

The responsibility for the fat ripoff is often shared by the service or product provider and the client. You, the client, may have done little or no self-assessment as to exactly what you are looking for in a program, what you truly need or what may be beneficial to your desired change, what priority you are willing to give your effort, or how realistic your expectations for the program are. You may only know intellectually that you want to be thin. The provider may be satisfied to offer exciting possibilities (illusions) simply because that is what you are looking for.

If I hear a client repeatedly refer to the program in the following manner, I know he or she is not prepared to evaluate the program objectively:

"Will 'it' take more than six months?"

"Has 'it' been effective with most people?"

Questions of this nature, which focus on "it" rather than individual efforts to change, clearly point out a search for magic. Of course, you can easily get your emotions and hopes raised by friends who are thin, by nationally publicized programs or aids, and misleading ads and book titles. The more elevated your emotions are, the less objective your decisions will be. Even if you have been ripped off several times previously, hope springs eternal, and when you're vainly straining to find magic, it is easy to mistake fool's gold for the real thing.

In the U.S., we seem to popularize, with the help of the media, several new magic weight-loss methods or diets every year. So, you, the overweight person, feeling emotionally stressed, rationalize that "If even a few of the stories about the new wonder plan are true, why couldn't 'it' work for me!?"

It is the same when you know someone who loses a substantial amount of weight. Do you stop to ask: "Am I different than that person?" "Was it water, lean muscle, or fat that was lost?" "Was the method used dangerous?" "How long has the weight been off?" The questions you're most likely to ask in this situation are, "How long did it take?" "How much did it cost?" and "Where can I get it?"

AVOID THE RIPOFF

If you are emotionally ready for another fat ripoff, you don't stop to notice if the content of a book is the same old story in new wrappings. Did the writer just coin a few new words and phrases? Is the diet just another diuretic diet made up of a different combination of foods and eating factors? Is the book full of motivational stories about the success of others, or endless weight loss recipes and pictures of pretty people in different exercise positions? None of these things will change *you*.

When you are considering a new weight-loss effort, you can avoid being ripped off by (1) securing the opinions of second and third parties who are knowledgeable and able to be objective about you and the program; (2) by being calm and taking your time when making a decision; (3) by checking on the background of the provider or the products; and (4) by determining if you will be required to make changes in yourself, your lifestyle, attitudes, and values.

The commercial weight-loss market offers some good, sound programs — and lots of fat ripoffs. The ripoffs sell best because they offer the easiest solutions to your weight problem. When you feel desperate, you simply want to close your eyes and wish for the magic to come true. As hard as it may be to believe, you may be one of those persons who make the fat ripoff programs and gimmicks possible. If you are in a constant quest for magic to save you from yourself, you become a likely target for the fat ripoffs.

> **"Help me doctor, but don't ask me to do anything that isn't quick, entertaining, painless, and cheap!"**

These are not the exact words used by any of the clients I have worked with during the past seven years; but in essence, it is the underlying cry of a great many overweight persons seeking magic answers.

In working with many individuals and groups and doing an in-depth research experiment, it was possible for me to have an ongoing dialogue with overweight people who spoke of strong desires to achieve attractive and healthy weight levels. We reviewed all of their previous efforts to control their weight. Diets by the score, fat clubs and gimmicks of all types had been used with little or no long-term success.

In my initial interviews with the overweight clients, determination, commitment, and optimism ran high. If they could just receive a little boost and some attention, they knew that they could make it (this time). *This* effort would be different. They "could not go on like this any longer." *"Things* had to change."

Most of the new clients had lengthy explanations as to why they had come to this point and why earlier efforts had not worked out: circumstances were never right; their parents taught them wrong; their spouse encouraged fatness; they had inherited it; they had a low metabolism; they were bored; they gained weight just by looking at food. Always a rationalization so as not to blame themselves. When overweight people were told that the programs for which they were applying held no magic and would take time, effort, and energy, they readily agreed to the challenge. They knew that their success depended upon themselves. They had already tried everything else, with no success. When the new clients were questioned about their willingness to change attitudes and values over a six-month period of time, again they agreed. However, they had one big question during the interviews, which dealt with the new electric shock machine. "Does it work?" they would ask with eager eyes. "Will it hurt me?" "When can I try it?" They would agree to long-term diet, exercise, group meetings, reading texts, changing activities, habit patterns, and so on — anything — just let them try that magic machine!

As potentially helpful as faradic therapy (electro-stimulus behavioral conditioning in which a shock is applied to the subject when he shows a desire for an "improper" food) can be for some people, it cannot, by itself, readjust eating patterns. It assists in getting rid of "hang-up" non-nutritious eating, and it helps to break such associations as TV and snacking. However, eating is necessary to life, and even nutritious food can be fattening. The overweight person is easily able to find new hang-up foods after extinguishing desire for an old one, which could mean a never-ending chase.

As a researcher, I soon became aware that the volunteer subjects were still counting on the magic and held clear aversions to real change in their lifestyles. Subjects seldom missed faradic therapy sessions, but often neglected to do exercises or attend group meetings. Staying on a balanced diet was very difficult for most, and attempting to use self-management conditioning techniques at home was next to impossible. The energy they were willing to put out for what they viewed as the magic answer was much greater than what they were willing to put out for the standard methods.

The greater effort to be consistent with the faradic therapy sessions (magic) did pay off for many people on a short-term basis. *Believing* a technique will work is a big part of its success. The clients would go along for weeks assuming they had built up an aversion to certain hang-up foods for which they had received the faradic shock therapy. It was then common for them to become curious about what would happen if they tried the food they thought they had an aversion to. About ten percent of the clients reported feeling nauseous, tense, or somehow aware of my voice saying they shouldn't eat that food, and they would, therefore, stay away from it. The other ninety percent quickly realized that no physical or mental aversion or conditioning had actually taken place — they were free to eat the hang-up food as usual. As more weeks and months passed, most of the ten percent that had experienced a negative association with their hang-up food found the psychological aversion had faded.

THE FOCUS IS ON YOU

All this effort for magic was not, however, without value. In the continuing group and individual discussions, the clients came to understand on an emotional level, as a result of their experiences, that for awhile, *as long as they* **believed** *the magic would work, it* **did** *work.* They did lose interest in the hang-up food for awhile. Now they knew at an emotional level, not just intellectually, that if they put the same effort and belief in *themselves,* the exercise and changing of food preferences would come about in the manner they desired. They now believed they could change.

They didn't need to waste time looking for any more magic — they could look to themselves. This was a change of focus from the **outside** to the **inside.**

Some of the clients may have come to this realization on their own, without aversion therapy, and others may not have. It was, however, openly discussed, and self-awareness grew with reinforcement from me, other staff members, and other clients.

Any magic illusion that has been uncovered can serve in this same way. Usually, however, the user of the magic that did not work feels foolish, disillusioned, angry, and cheated. But, the worst part is that disillusioned people may feel less capable of changing their condition and give up or become easy prey for the next magic cure.

Once the aversion therapy clients had changed their focus, it still did not mean their troubles were over. They still needed to learn to believe in themselves through their own efforts. Each person still had exercise to do, attitudes to change, new food preferences to develop. Learning to believe in yourself and making lifestyle changes does not happen in one lesson.

The chronically overweight person has tremendous fears, guilt, and anxiety about his feelings of inadequacy — feelings that seem overpowering. People without a weight problem often find it hard to empathize and tend to put down those overweight people going through what is frequently a struggle of desperation.

While holding supportive individual discussion sessions, it became apparent that basic attitudes and values were what needed changing. These overweight people had the same frustrations with marriage, children, job, and sexuality as other people. However, their frustrations led to inappropriate eating. Food represented security, entertainment, comfort, sensual gratification, reward, and achievement. If long-term weight control was to come about, the whole person had to be examined. Difficult change had to take place in many aspects of the overweight person's life. A positive self-image needed to be developed. A self-improving effort needed to be made in many areas for a long enough period that the obese person learned to *prefer* self-improving ways of living and eating. Then it would not be necessary to continually suppress inappropriate, self-defeating behavior.

For an overweight person who came looking for magic, these ideas were very heavy and hard to face. With a great deal of support and encouragement on the part of myself and the other therapists, albeit not without pain, confusion, depression, and anger on the part of the overweight subjects, many positive changes and self-improving moves were made toward a healthy, slim way of life. No magic could do what had to be done, and it was not always easy or fun. However, when the quest for magic was extinguished, new energy to *work* became available.

When the overweight person came to realize and accept the idea that there was no magic and that only his own motivation, effort, responsibility, and decision could bring about needed changes, the question arose: "Do I really want to change?" If the answer was "yes," positive change came (with effort); and the more change that came about, the easier it became. If the answer was "no" or "I don't know," the negative fat condition continued. A clear decision to change had to be made. The hope for outside magic to save them had to then be given up.

The overweight subjects were given support in their positive efforts and were facilitated in becoming aware of their choices, but the pain and effort was theirs. **The magic (better known as freedom) was within each person.** A place to go, people who cared, aversion conditioning, weight measurement and monitoring, relaxation training, counseling, group support, lectures, literature, and self-management training all gave helpful backing, but each person who successfully made it did so without outside magic, and that was his or her real success — to know the magic was on the inside all the time, in the form of new self-confidence and improved self-image.

Although searching for outside magic usually ends in disappointment, poorer self-image, and greater pain or more fat, people only seem to let go of the quest at four points:

1. **When the boredom gets so great it seems as if there is nothing else to do.**
2. **When the physical or emotional pain is so great it seems that there is no choice.**
3. **When the quest seems so hopeless, and they feel so helpless, there is nothing else to do.**
4. **When the overweight person simply realizes that he or she is free to change.**

Straining to change can be counterproductive. When clients relaxed and assumed changes would come about — while making consistent efforts — success was theirs. When you let go of the struggle to force things to happen and make a relaxed, consistent effort, the changes come easier and faster.

Are you ready to give up the search for outside magic to save you? Now? The fear of letting go can be great because the unknown lies ahead, but the pain and fear of staying the same is even worse.

6

THE HIDDEN FEARS OF BECOMING THIN

Because my weight-loss programs focus a great deal on emotions, I wish to make it very clear at the start of this chapter that the people I see as clients are relatively stable — part of that great middle group of average people. A small number of this group may be highly emotionally stressed at times, but rarely do I see anyone who could be classified as "mentally ill."

Although I fully acknowledge the important role and influence that heredity, organic illness or injury, cultural conditioning, sedentary lifestyle, poor nutritional education, and economic, work, and living conditions play in chronic weight problems, it is unusual to find a person who eats compulsively (inappropriately) who is eating out of hunger. According to my experience and research, it is much more the rule that the person who eats excessively is responding to an emotional reaction, i.e. loneliness, fear, boredom, anxiety, excitement, etc., and would really like to be close to someone and be comforted — "hugged" — "touched." Food is sensual. We react to it by sight, taste, and smell. After opening the refrigerator twenty times, why not give in and trade off one sensual need — touching — for a substitute — tasty food.

People commonly use food as a means of attempting to deal with their emotional needs. Sometimes it is obvious and clear to the food abuser, and other times it is hidden or suppressed. To help classify yourself in this respect, complete the following quiz to see if you are an "emotional eater."

THE EMOTIONAL EATING QUIZ

Answering True or False, indicate which of the following you do three or more times each week. Score 10 points for each true answer.

1. Eat more when lonely, excited, anxious, fearful, bored, angry, depressed, etc. _____
2. Put food away in unusual places for later use. _____
3. Eat large volumes of food when alone and small amounts when you are with other people. _____
4. Approach your food preparation as an artist would his drawings, or spend a great deal of time planning ahead for meals as special events. _____
5. Use the food interest of friends, relatives, spouse, or others as a means of, or an excuse for, getting the type and volume of food you want. _____
6. Have two or more alcoholic beverages in a day. _____
7. Dream of foods you want, or have nightmares involving food and eating. _____
8. Feel self-conscious about how your body looks. _____
9. Eat foods you know are bad for you, and then feel rebellious or guilty. _____
10. Continue to eat after your stomach has clearly registered full. _____
11. Use drugs to suppress appetite, to put you to sleep, to wake you up, to keep you calm, etc. _____
12. Struggle with internal conflicts about dieting, exercise, or the effect of your weight on your health, appearance, and achievement. _____
13. Pay attention to, or get interested in, commercial ads about magic weight-loss methods and beautiful, youthful bodies. _____
14. Have fantasies about what it would be like to be thinner or fatter. _____
15. Feel resentment, prejudice, or envy towards people who are big eaters and still have an evenly balanced body. _____

YOUR SCORE	THE LIKELIHOOD OF EATING AS AN ADJUSTMENT REACTION TO YOUR EMOTIONS
130 - 150	**Extremely high.** Counseling strongly advised.
100 - 120	**Very high.** Counseling suggested.
80 - 90	**High.** Evaluation for counseling could prove helpful.
60 - 70	**Moderate.** Support group or classes, self-awareness, and conscious effort advised.
10 - 50	**Unlikely.** Classes, self-awareness, and personal desire could prove useful.
0	**Low.** Involvement with food is in balance with emotional needs.

Nutritional education and exercise program is advised for all.

A score of one hundred or more may indicate a need for professional help in coming to understand your feelings and finding more effective adjustments to them. If you are a chronically overweight person with a score of eighty or more, you are not likely to lose your extra pounds and keep them off without becoming more self-aware and dealing more directly with your concerns.

The *Emotional Eating Quiz* is a cursory check on the degree of emotional involvement you have with your eating habits. Considering other variables such as basal metabolic rate (BMR), exercise or lack of it, food choices, etc., a high score (one hundred or more) may not necessarily indicate that you will become obese or even overweight. Bulemics (bingers who eat huge amounts of food and then use vomiting or laxatives to get rid of what they ate) and anorexics (those who experience chronic fear of appetite for food) require testing far beyond the limited elements considered in this brief quiz.

Evaluating Your Answers

Considering all of these questions except #4, if any of your true responses indicate in excess of three or more times a week, or on a continuous basis over several months, just a single true answer may be reason enough to seek out a qualified professional assessment.

Answering true to questions #1, 2, 3, 5, 9, and 10 indicate that you have a greater need to fulfill than simply satisfying nature's hunger call. To answer true to these questions may indicate food is being used to comfort and soothe emotional feelings, or it is being used to distract from them.

Answering true to questions #6 or 11 may indicate the potential development of a habit that could lead to an addiction, which could include food abuse or having feelings of a loss of control or dependency.

Answering true to questions #8, 12, 14, and 15 is more an indication of negative feelings about your body, its fat, and what it represents to your self-image and social inter-actions. Feeling uncomfortable about your body can lead to depressed feelings that may in turn lead to a greater need for sensual comforting from food, which in turn can lead to more fat.

Answering true to #4 may indicate a preoccupation with food as security in relationships. Using food to manipulate, or using food preparation as a means of gaining approval or praise, of feeling worthy or needed, is usually done by a spouse who feels insecure in the marriage relationship.

Answering true to #7 may be an indication of restricted drives for the emotional fulfillment you think food can offer, self-defeating behavior you desire, or guilt about your waking activities with food and fat.

Answering true to #13 may relate to a desire to be saved from yourself, while feeling weak and out of control where food is concerned. It may also relate to a fear of facing reality regarding weight loss and/or eating habits. You may have any one of a number of reasons for not wanting to become self-aware, or not wanting to discover why you may feel a need to stay overweight, when consciously you want to be thin.

FAT IS A SYMPTOM

I find overweight people to be like other people, except their stress, fears, and feelings of inadequacy are realized as the symptom of fat. People who are hyperactive and skinny, the compulsive smoker, those who take too many drinks or drugs, the type "A" high blood pressure sufferer, those who suffer from nervous skin conditions and organic breakdowns of one type or another, are all potentially the victims of stress and ineffective adjustments in attempting to deal with the same types of stress, fears, and feelings of inadequacy evidenced by the symptom of fat with the overweight person.

With the chronically overweight person, it is most common to suppress awareness of one or more of the feelings that produce the symptom of fat. These suppressed feelings are most apt to be fears — fears of what would happen if the extra pounds were to be lost; thus, internal conflict exists. Consciously, the overweight person sees every logical reason for and benefit of being thin; however, on a suppressed, unaware level, the same person is apt to be fearful of what becoming thin represents.

The fear of becoming thin could be as simple as giving up one's sensual friend (food), which has been there to give that extra comfort whenever it was needed, or it could be as involved as threatening the stability of a marriage.

CASE HISTORIES

The following case histories show examples of the role inner fears and feelings can play in being overweight:

Case #1. Mary quickly became overweight shortly after her marriage ten years ago. She had married more out of a need for security than for love. Her husband, who felt insecure about himself, had a deep fear of being alone, and was possessive and jealous of Mary. His jealousy came out as criticism. This criticism upset Mary because it represented a threat to the security of her marriage. She sought comfort, and with no one to turn to, feeling inadequate and alone, she found her comfort in food. As she quickly gained weight, her husband's criticism stopped. Evidently he felt no threat of losing Mary as long as she was overweight. Mary and her husband were unable to have children, which was very disappointing to her. She felt that children would fulfill her need to be needed and loved. Eventually, Mary took a part-time job and learned marketable job skills, all along claiming the desire to be a full-time housewife and mother. The more capable of earning a living she became, the more angry she became inside, and the more critical of the world. She began to have fantasies of being thin again, as well as being promiscuous, something she had always feared and considered to be morally wrong.

As it turned out, after a few months in a safe, supportive growth group, Mary was able to identify her inner fears:

1. She was angry at her husband for wanting her to stay fat so he wouldn't be jealous and leave her; if she let her anger out, it also threatened her marriage.

2. If she became thin, her fantasy about promiscuity would come true, which would end her marriage. (Promiscuity represented a means of getting back at the one who controlled her while demonstrating her attractiveness.)

3. Her expectation of herself as a "Good" housewife and mother would be lost. She'd never be loved or secure again.

Case #2. Joe was 5'7" tall and weighed in at three hundred + pounds. He had a friendly, likeable manner, and thus was well thought of in his community. He was very skilled at his work and had established a flourishing business. Joe's doctor had told him that he must either lose weight or risk premature death. Joe had strong conflicting feelings, in that he consciously wanted to lose the extra pounds so he could live long enough to see his kids grow up; yet his emotions seemed to keep him eating far beyond his physical needs. He felt confused, torn, and frustrated.

During counseling, Joe realized that at the relatively short stature of 5'7", much of his perception of his masculinity was wrapped up in his three-hundred + pounds. As he said, "If I lose weight, nobody will notice me coming; at this weight, everybody does!" He felt that he could even lose his business. "My size is part of my identity — it makes me special." The fear of losing weight was greater than keeping the weight on and risking death, and he had not even realized it. His fears of early death or losing his masculine image (his identity) were emotions which made the desire for comfort from food even greater.

Case #3. Joyce taught school for one year before having two children and spending the next fifteen years at home. During this time, her weight fluctuated often, but gradually worked upward far beyond her ideal weight of one-hundred-ten pounds. Joyce felt unfulfilled as a housewife, and knew her family could use extra income in preparation for the children's college educations. Also, she felt that her husband, although he didn't complain, had shown less sexual interest in her and was beginning to look more at shapelier women.

After being a housewife all those years, Joyce knew her teaching skills were possibly no longer adequate. She felt that with the stiff competition for positions she'd never be hired, even if she updated her skills, because she would be competing with younger, trimmer, and more attractive candidates. Also, she'd feel embarrassed to appear on campus for the refresher classes she needed, carrying all that extra weight. She must lose the fat first. But somehow, that never seemed to happen, and she felt confused. Why couldn't she drop those pounds?

Joyce was a person who had become paranoid about her abilities to compete and the possibility of failure. With her rationale, she would never face failure on the job, since her handicap, **"FAT,"** would keep her safe from making an effort. If she did make a try (while fat) and failed, she would have a good excuse. Her paranoia about the work world was greater than her fear of not having money for the children's education or the loss of her husband's sexual interest.

These are typical examples of people having fears of becoming thin and rationalizing or suppressing them, while they look for magic cures outside themselves that will never come. When these same people look into themselves in a supportive, safe environment, they find their own answers.

In my programs at John C. Lincoln Hospital in Phoenix, Arizona, I certainly adhere to the usual practical weight-loss methods of good nutrition, balanced exercise, relaxation training, behavioral conditioning techniques, testing, etc. However, I feel that individual and group counseling must be utilized to identify and resolve those hidden fears and feelings in order for long term weight management (two, five, ten years down the road) to be assured. Learning to practice self-awareness and face fears that have prevented resolution of weight problems will also provide the assertiveness and self-confidence necessary to be consistent with healthy diet and exercise habits.

FACING THE FEARS THAT ARE KEEPING YOU FAT

To discover ulterior or subconscious motives about yourself requires a great deal of open, honest objectivity. This is very hard to do when you examine yourself, because you are only on the inside looking out. You have your ego to protect. It is hard enough to like yourself when you're fat; to learn that you may be *deliberately* keeping yourself fat for some negative reason could be overwhelming. So, why not just tuck those bad possibilities away and forget them?

> **Because, to hide from yourself gives you more reason to dislike yourself than any reason you have for staying fat.**

Your potential is also a huge unknown, so you are missing a part of your identity. But unknowns are very anxiety producing. When you have anxiety you seek comfort, which may often be in the sensual form of food — which in turn gives you more fat about which to be unhappy. Round and round it goes, and where it stops only you can know.

To change all this requires letting down your defenses and acknowledging that an emotion is the driving cause for self-defeating eating. You are dealing with a fear, so letting down defenses takes courage. *Did you ever think that if you were never afraid you'd have no chance to be brave?* If you see yourself as being brave, you have a reason to like yourself. People usually ask me at this point, "Well, how do I let my defenses down?" One way is to open up to the fear itself on your own initiative. If someone *pushes* you toward your fear, your defenses and fear become greater. If a person has a fear of water and thinks he can't swim, we know it won't help to push him off the deep end, as he could panic and drown. As stated earlier, when you decide to approach your fears — on your own initiative — you should do so gradually, so you don't overwhelm yourself. You need to go through a desensitization process, taking one step at a time toward what you fear, holding your ground until you are comfortable with where you are. Then take as many steps toward the fear as possible until discomfort is experienced, where again you hold your ground until you are comfortable. Again, on you go until all of the fear is extinguished. It may be necessary to approach the fear only in your fantasy and become comfortable with that first, before testing reality.

Because it is very hard for any of us to see ourselves clearly enough to identify our fears, feedback and constructive criticism from outside are useful. Generally, each person sees you from a different perspective, and yet, if you get the honest views of many people who know you, you can probably find some opinions that are held in common. Then you can begin to see yourself from the outside in.

If you are going to collect open, honest opinions that have value, you need people who have known you in different situations and for different lengths of time; people who have given you some attention and who value you enough to give you their time, observations, and feelings. If you are a part of an encounter Gestalt group, it will be easy to get some feedback, but you need it from other sources too. In any case, the best way I know to get it is to give it. You gain another person's trust and openness by offering yours. Sometimes you won't get it at all, but most of the time you'll get the same amount of trust you offer. When you have this general kind of exchange, you'll come to understand where your fears are, and thus, your ulterior or subconscious motives for staying fat.

LETTING DOWN YOUR DEFENSES

What you are doing in establishing this open exchange with people is building a bridge of trust. As you do this trust building, the more safe you begin to feel, and the more you are able to drop your defenses, enabling your subconscious fears to come to the surface. Discovering your hidden fear or motivations for staying overweight is a matter of stimulating your own acceptance of those fears by relaxing your defenses, as you do when you feel safe. Notice that all the methods mentioned here attempt, in some way, to bring about a safe feeling in you.

> **The safer you feel, the more you will drop your defenses.**

Self-hypnosis and meditation are other means of learning your ulterior or subconscious purposes. Intense concentration while relaxed will aid all of your efforts. Even when you are seeking feedback from others, if you will relax yourself first with a method such as yoga, you'll find your exchange with others easier and more profitable.

To learn self-hypnosis, meditation, or yoga, it is a good idea to read reference books on the subjects and attend classes. Usually it is easy to find inexpensive classes at local YMCA'S, adult education evening courses, colleges, and high schools. Learning these methods of relaxation (letting defenses down) is useful in other ways too, but none of them will help unless you actually incorporate them into your lifestyle.

USE YOUR DREAMS

Once you have mastered a relaxation technique (see Chapter 9 for detailed information), you may wish to utilize your dreams as a means of seeking out your subconscious motives. Prior to getting into bed, relax yourself as completely as possible. When this is accomplished, permit yourself to have a mental image of yourself sleeping deeply. When your image is clear, suggest to yourself over and over that you will remember your dream this night, and that you will write down on a paper what you dreamed the moment you awaken.

Practice this routine for a few weeks or until you have been successful several times in recalling your dreams. The next step then is to not only suggest to yourself that you'll remember your dreams, but also that you will dream about your fear of losing your weight. Continue to repeat these suggestions until they are realized. It aids your pre-sleep suggestions at night to also make the same suggestions to yourself many times during the day. When you suggest to yourself that you will remember your fears during your dream, also suggest that the dream will not upset you; that you will remain calm when you confront your fear.

DEAL WITH YOUR FEARS

The last step is dealing with the fear you have confronted. You can use the desensitization method described for you earlier, or you can continue to work with your dreams until you realize that you are dreaming at the time you are dreaming. When you are aware that you're dreaming during the time of your dream, you can do whatever you like in that dream. Place your fear in some type of symbolic form such as a package or a ball. When you are sure your fear is contained in a ball, kill it. Blow it up, burn it, shoot it full of holes; do whatever you like, but destroy it in your dream, and relief from it will result in reality.

The possible ulterior or subconscious motives people may have for staying fat are infinite. I hesitate to mention any specifically, as I don't want them to serve as suggestions with which you can identify or limit yourself. Nor do I want you to respond to them quickly with your defenses up. If your defenses are up, and I hit a button (fear), your defenses could go even higher with rationalizations and denial.

By the way, the brighter a person is, the more clever he or she can be at rationalizing. As indicated in the case histories outlined in this chapter, one possible ulterior or subconscious reason for staying fat is that the fat person *wants* a handicap. "If everyone knows I am handicapped, they won't expect as much from me, and thus, I have fewer chances to fail." Is it safest to be fat? As I said, the possibilities are unlimited. Are you brave enough and ready enough to start looking good?

In my programs we are constantly looking for these hidden fears — the very sensitive, emotional buttons you have been avoiding. Whether you are aware of your emotional buttons and are deliberately avoiding them, or if the fears have been pushed into your subconscious, the need is the same. That is, to bring them up in front and keep them there until they are resolved.

If you should feel these methods are not for you, psychoanalysis or psychotherapy are other options available. Most people who seek these types of assistance are *not* "crazy." They're only people trying to improve their lives.

7

PROCRASTINATION

A WAY TO AVOID BEING THIN

When Sue entered my weight-loss program, she was action oriented. During our three month contact, she sought and found self-awareness, utilized program offerings, and fit what she learned into her existing busy schedule. She quickly made adjustments in an open minded, non-resisting manner and her desired changes came about. With new information she gained new value preferences and lost the undesired pounds. The whole process went almost unbelievably smoothly, for a number of reasons: Sue was only thirty pounds overweight, and with a comparatively easy goal, she saw a good chance for success; she was an ex-smoker and a dry alcoholic with strong religious beliefs. Because of past experience with successful change, she had ample reason to believe she could achieve her desired goal.

All these factors contributed to Sue's smooth progress — progress most clients only dream about. As a result of her background experiences, she had learned some very hard lessons, among them the ability to overcome the tendency to *procrastinate*. Sue had learned to take the *action* necessary to solve a problem and effect a change.

Procrastination is a common character trait that is found in the young and old, rich and poor, strong and weak, male and female. Almost everyone puts off doing what needs to be done at some point in his life, and it seems especially common among those people entering weight-loss programs. People like Sue are truly exceptional. For those seeking permanent weight changes, dealing with tendencies to procrastinate is not only common, but also of primary importance.

As I mentioned in Chapter 5, only ten percent of those who depend on assistance with weight reduction have long-term success. One possible reason for this situation is that some of the ninety percent who do not achieve their goal sabotage their own effort, and one way of doing this is by procrastination.

As a therapist with the task of facilitating change in others, I have no bigger challenge than helping develop motivation to overcome the habit of procrastination. Even for those who have the motivation to learn to let go of procrastination, the process is not simple, clear, or easy. Procrastination may not prove to be self-defeating, self-depreciating, or harmful in all cases, but to the person who is trying to lose weight it is *deadly*. To the seriously overweight person, procrastination means emotional pain, physical discomfort, lost opportunities, social embarrassment, loss of time, money, self esteem, and worst of all, health. Under these circumstances, the wisdom of letting go of procrastination is without logical challenge.

Among those people who do not see themselves as procrastinators, there is a tendency to moralize — to label procrastination as "laziness," "lack of discipline," or "bad habits." Some people like to believe it is just a matter of being unorganized, and if they could only learn to manage their time more effectively, the procrastination would end; however, somehow they just keep postponing that time management class or put off getting their management plan into operation. In my experience, I have found that moralizing blame only produces additional guilt to pile upon the already existing guilt and feelings of inadequacy experienced by procrastinators. Also the teaching of time management and behavioral techniques for the procrastinator to implement on his own only offers something more about which to procrastinate or feel guilty about not doing — which is why so many diet plans and recipes have been lost in the dust of cupboards around the world.

PROCRASTINATION OFTEN MEANS FEAR

In my own life, as well as that of many of my clients, laziness, lack of willpower, bad habits, lack of discipline, or not knowing how to manage time is *not* the cause of procrastination. In fact, many of the procrastinators I have worked with have been highly organized, compulsive perfectionists and workaholics, with tremendous supplies of willpower to avoid, rationalize, and put off logical choices. The more exact cause of procrastination is difficult to "understand" because it is not an intellectual problem, but rather an emotional one. It is most often a *fear* that has been developed slowly from childhood or suppressed because of feelings of inadequacy and weak egos. In most instances I have encountered, procrastination serves as protection from fears or provides some type of reward or secondary gain. Commonly the procrastinator is either not aware of his deeper feelings or he is choosing to ignore or suppress this awareness.

Carlos, an aerospace engineer, was a highly organized perfectionist. He was creative, bright, and sensitive, and had always been a very giving person. But Carlos had been very lonely since his divorce. He faithfully attended group meetings, took notes, and acted on suggestions to which he could comfortably relate. The action and notes were to be part of his GRAND PLAN to start a diet and exercise program that somehow never happened.

He gradually realized that he was procrastinating and became frustrated when he couldn't understand why he was putting off doing what he thought he sincerely wanted to do.

In individual counseling sessions, we came to understand that Carlos had always been a gentle giver and a doer for others as a means of obtaining friends. His need to please others was often greater than his need to please himself. In his mind, what he could "do" for others was the only thing that gave him worth. When, in group counseling, he became aware of this, he began to let go of many one-way friendships. Now, without "doing" for others, he felt that he had little or nothing to offer, and if he lost weight and was rejected, he would know for sure that he was worthless as a person. When he gave away his engineering skills in return for friendships that weren't fulfilling, his skills were the worth that made him acceptable. Weighing one-hundred extra pounds meant that he had to "give" to compensate for his defect. Without his extra pounds to blame, it would be just Carlos "the person" and rejection would be devastating, so why chance it? The risk was too great. Procrastinate.

Once Carlos let down his defenses in counseling he quickly identified and understood his fear of rejection and of not having worth as a person. He saw that it was not a matter of finding the right diet or exercise plan. Although self-awareness gave him options and some relief from his frustrations, awareness alone did not stop the procrastinating. He still had to face his fears.

Although self-awareness is essential to long-term, effective change, it is still only a starting place in the process of change. Procrastination *served* Carlos and *frustrated* him at the same time. The fear or secondary gain that went with procrastination was still there to be dealt with.

Procrastination helps avoid fears of such things as:

* **Success** — I won't be able to handle it. People will expect me to keep it up. My friends will reject me or may even be angry with me for doing better than they are.
* **Guilt** — I'm not worthy of the benefits of being thin.

* **Self-esteem** — I'll find out I'm not as good as every-one says I should be.
* **New challenges** — If I lose the handicap of my extra weight, I will be expected to try things I don't have to try now, and I'll fail.
* **Standing out in the crowd** — People attack those who stand out, and I'll be noticed as different and rejected.
* **I'll be promiscuous** — If I lose weight, attractive men (or women) will want me and all those fantasies I've had will come true.
* **The unknown** — If I change, all kinds of things may happen that I can't deal with.
* **Loss of specialness** — My size gets me notice and attention that I'll lose if I'm thin.

Some rewards or secondary gains that procrastination provides:

* **Revenge** — a passive-aggressive way of getting back at others who are a source of my anger or hurt.
* **Rebellion** — a way of showing authority figures they can't control me or force me to lose weight.
* **Power** — a means of controlling others. The word "no" can mean power.
* **Pressure to act** — procrastination puts on a last minute pressure so that I can get by with doing the minimum of what is expected.
* **Magic** — if I wait long enough, someone or something will save me and I'll know I'm loved the way I am, and I can avoid the pain of change.

People wanting to lose weight or overcome procrastina-tion are frequently the same in that they are not too interested in the *cause* of their problem. They are much more interested in *how* to change. This is again a search for quick, easy "magic."

When we wish for things to "happen" to us quickly, without effort, and if by chance these things do occur, the insight and experience we should have gained is missing and it postpones the real achievement of the goal: letting go of procrastination.

MOTIVATION – PROCRASTINATION

Now that possible reasons for procrastination have been discussed, you are aware of how self-defeating it can be. The next logical step should be to let go of procrastination. However, I feel it would be valuable at this point to look briefly at motivation — the topic of the following chapter — as it relates to procrastination. Motivation and procrastination may at first seem to be in a chicken-and-egg situation, that is, it is hard to tell which came first. Upon closer examination, it becomes clear that procrastination requires motivation. It requires motivation to either maintain procrastination or to let it go. As I have already pointed out, fear and reward are usually root causes of procrastination. They are also the motivation which keeps procrastination alive. This prerequisite does not apply in reverse. Procrastination is likely to inhibit motivation.

At the same time, both procrastination and motivation are integral parts of the problem of losing weight and developing a healthful, self-enhancing lifestyle. What enables a person to let go of procrastination is apt to serve in the development of motivation. Motivation builds on itself and to let go of procrastination requires motivation, among other things.

Determining the cause of procrastination is necessary to long-term change, but just possessing this information will not, in itself, bring about change. Rather, some motivation to change and the opportunity to be more accurate and realistic in attacking the problem is necessary. Carlos felt support from the group. He was praised for his small efforts and subjected to very little pressure by their expectations for him, which prompted him to lay out some of his well-organized plans. Making his plans known to the group provided the extra motivation of a small degree of social pressure. He knew, however, that if he didn't come through, these people would still be supportive and would encourage him to try again.

Carlos also lowered his expectations of himself; he did not strain for perfection, but rather worked towards small improvements in his consistency to change his diet and to exercise regularly. He also involved himself in a food co-op where he did not let his engineering skills be known; therefore, he could not rely on using these skills to win friends. As he began working and being involved with new people on a new basis, he also began to realize he could be liked for his values, ideas, and personality — in other words for himself. When he saw that he could be accepted and appreciated in spite of being overweight and without resorting to one-way giving, he began to view himself differently. He began to believe that he no longer needed the excuse of his weight; that he no longer needed to justify paying for friendships with his skills; he no longer needed to protect himself from finding out if he would be a lovable person in a trim body.

The following information derived from Carlos's experience may be of use to you:

1. Establish a support system in which you feel safe enough to confront fears of changing.
2. In the safe environment, with defenses down, it is possible to acknowledge procrastination and

develop the insight to see and accept the underlying causes of procrastination (fears).

3. Reassess personal values and define new, flexible directions for future development, seeking new potentials (motivation).
4. Lower expectations of perfection to more realistic goals.
5. Facilitate motivation with self-awareness and appreciation of small successes and development of new skills.

Beyond what Carlos did in his effort to let go of procrastination, here are additional steps you can take:

6. Develop skill in any relaxation technique, such as self-hypnosis, meditation, or biofeedback — building confidence for other more threatening changes.
7. Use behavioral techniques, such as contracts, which provide rewards or punishments (rewards work better).
8. Organize a group where you facilitate and model behavior. "We learn most when we teach."
9. Work out unresolved conflicts with others you care about (especially important with authority figures).
10. Use the desensitization process in confronting fears.
11. Learn to stimulate your senses and imagery skills.

If you can realize that there is more discomfort and disappointment in remaining a procrastinator than in becoming action-oriented and facing fears, the whole process of change will seem more inviting.

8

I'd Be Thin If Only I Could Get Motivated!

When Nancy, a small boned, five foot, one-hundred sixty-pound woman complained about the extra pounds she couldn't seem to lose, I asked her the usual questions, including questions about exercise. She replied, "Yes, I have a regular exercise routine." I exercise with Richard Simmons while I watch his TV program every morning."

Trying not to sound skeptical, I pursued the exercise aspect of Nancy's weight-loss efforts. Her responses were mostly soft spoken, but full of defensive protests and a great many qualifications and rationalizations that were laden with guilt feelings:

* She had never been athletic.
* Her husband didn't exercise.
* She was so busy with her children.
* She had tried group exercise with her neighbors several times, but they always quit after a short time.

Therefore, the only thing left was to rely on Richard Simmons.

Nancy was really saying three things: (1) I feel guilty for not being in better shape, and it's obvious and embarrassing, since everybody can see I'm fat; (2) I think I'm lazy, and that makes me a bad person; (3) I need to get motivated from outside — my friends, neighbors, my husband, or Richard Simmons — I can't motivate myself to do anything about my body.

Nancy's feelings about herself are common among overweight people, even though they may be highly motivated in other aspects of their lives. Many of us are caught up in self-defeating compulsions such as when we don't do what we know we are capable of, what is socially popular, or what we think is expected of us, we feel bad about ourselves, which makes it more difficult to change. We look for an excuse to justify our behavior, and "I can't get motivated" is a great one. Nobody can prove that it isn't true. Motivation is elusive and nebulous, making it impossible for *others* to find a satisfactory answer for us. We can even convince ourselves that we've made every effort to find that sure-fire motivator.

WHAT IS MOTIVATION?

Let's be brave and look at motivation. What is it? Where does it come from? According to my *Dictionary of Psychology: "**to motivate:** to incite to action — to serve as an incentive or goal; **motivation:** an intervening variable which is used to account for factors within the organism (you) which arouse, maintain, and channel behavior toward a goal; **motive:** a state of tension within the individual which arouses, maintains, and directs behavior toward a goal — the conscious or unconscious reason for behavior — the drive, set, or attitude which guides behavior."*[1]

Among psychologists, the concept of motive (or motivation) is one of the most controversial — with a great many theories and definitions. The concept is also laden with the connotations and overtones of many other commonly used English terms such as appetite, attitude, desire, determination, drive, emotion, end, goal, habit, impulse, incentive, instinct, interest, need, preference, set, and sentiment.

[1]J.P. Chaplin, *Dictionary of Psychology* (New York, NY: Dell Publishing Co., 1968.)

Difficult, if not impossible, as it may be to define motivation or motive in a clear, precise, understandable manner, one thing does seem clear.

> **Motivation must come from within to be truly effective. Dependency on outside motivators almost always results in failure.**

Let's get back to Nancy. All of her life she had struggled to meet relationship and career goals which weren't achieved, she felt, due to her excess weight. Despite an avid study of weight loss diets and nutrition, the use of "magic gimmicks," neighborhood exercise groups, and memberships in an impressive roster of reducing clubs and dance classes, Nancy was still carrying around those extra pounds. She had had some temporary success with weight loss at one time through the use of diet pills, but along with the weight loss came the unpleasant side effects of nervousness, sleeplessness, and headaches.

Although I had explained to Nancy at our first session together that neither I nor my program held any magic cures for overweight, I could see that the fires of hope burned brightly, and they were hard to extinguish with words. The approach of my program was new to Nancy, and because it was different from anything she had tried previously, she was excited about the prospect of "it" making her thin.

Nancy attended all meetings regularly and with great eagerness. She was very open to trying all the various relaxation techniques, she shared her feelings about her desire for a career, her marriage, and her other family relationships. But even though she was following all the right moves, nothing was happening as far as weight loss. She was still waiting and hoping for the program, or me, or "it" to make her lose weight.

Finally, after having passed through stages of frustration, fright, and depression, Nancy arrived at a critical point. She began to really take a look at me, at the program, and most of all at herself. She realized that she had never given up the search for magic — the magic to make her do what she didn't think she could do herself. She became aware of the fact that she, and she alone, was responsible for herself and for her actions. Her focus turned inward as these revelations became clearer.

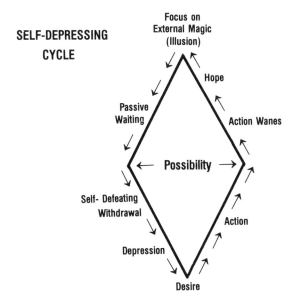

There is fear involved in looking inside yourself. It's much easier to look to external support for making decisions and taking action, and to blame external sources or circumstances in case of failure. But, as Nancy's focus turned inward, she became aware of herself as a person for the first time. She began to realize that SHE was the important element. That she needed to devote HER thoughts, time, and energy to achieving her goals. She established her priorities, and from these priorities, she developed her personal philosophy of life. She learned to identify what had meaning and purpose to her.

In the beginning, the realization and acceptance of self-responsibility was a heavy burden. It was frightening to Nancy to know that this "inadequate person" she had thought herself to be was in charge. But, gradually, the feeling of heavy responsibility was replaced with an exhilirating sense of freedom. Freedom to be who and what she chose to be; to explore courses of action, and to change those courses of action if they felt inappropriate. One step at a time she moved towards becoming the person she had hardly dared dream she could be. As shedding pounds became secondary to the goal of taking charge of her life, the weight began to come off almost without conscious effort. Nancy had made many successful changes in her life, and from these successes she learned to trust in her own abilities and decisions. Once she trusted herself to make decisions and to follow through with appropriate action, any goal was within her reach.

THE PATH TO SELF-MOTIVATION

The steps toward self-motivation which Nancy went through can be summarized as follows:

1. **DESIRE** — First there has to be the desire to achieve a goal, whatever it may be. In Nancy's case, she had the desire to lose weight, but she lacked the tools to enable her to act on her desire.
2. **POSSIBILITY** — Because Nancy had a desire — to lose weight — she was searching for possibilities. She saw my program as a possibility.
3. **HOPE** — The availability of a possible solution to Nancy's problem led to hope, and hope became the motivating force she could use to begin taking action.

SELF-CREATED MOTIVATION

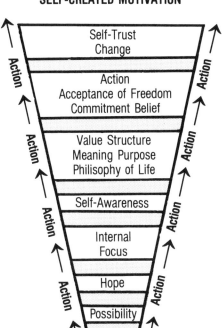

4. **INTERNAL FOCUS** — Once Nancy had accept-
    ed the fact that there WAS no external magic, she
    began to look inside herself and to draw on her own
    abilities and strengths.
5. **SELF-AWARENESS** — With her focus turned
    inward, Nancy began to get acquainted with herself.
    She became aware of herself as a person.
6. **PHILOSOPHY OF LIFE** — Self-awareness led to
    Nancy's prioritizing her values and determining
    what had real meaning and purpose in her life. This
    in turn led to the development of a personal
    philosophy of life which enabled her to make deci-
    sions in accordance with her beliefs.
7. **ACCEPTANCE OF FREEDOM** — At this point,
    Nancy was ready to accept the freedom of assuming

responsibility for herself and her actions. She *believed* she could handle this freedom and that she would be able to take the right actions.

8. **CHANGE** — Now, finally, Nancy was ready to make some real changes in herself and in her life.

9. **SELF-TRUST** — Because she had become aware of herself, had accepted her freedom, and had made successful changes, Nancy learned to trust herself. She had *earned* her belief in herself. She knew that whatever her goals in life were to be as she worked towards further self-improvement she now had the ability and strength to achieve those goals. She had developed confidence that she was in charge of herself and that she was able to create her own motivation.

Throughout all these steps, continuous *ACTION* is vital. Inaction kills the energy necessary to move forward.

Summary

It's easy to summarize the process Nancy went through. It is *not* easy to go through it. Most of the process is difficult, especially at first. But once you begin taking the steps toward developing self-motivational skills, you realize that it isn't something totally new. The difference is that now you've become aware of yourself and you're making deliberate decisions that are right for you and your life. Although some external stimuli (such as a support group) can be helpful as you work towards your goal, the true efforts must come from within. Finally you've realized that you don't need your husband, your friends, or Richard Simmons to motivate you to do what you really wanted to do all along. You have learned the skill of generating your own motivation.

9

THE STRESS FACTOR

A great many weight-loss programs do not attempt to deal with the fact, or even acknowledge, that stress (distress) can be a major factor in weight gain or loss. More than ample research, including my own, has been done which identifies stress as a major contributing factor in weight gain or loss, as well as many other counterproductive behaviors. Not only can obesity result from stress, but also, being overweight can contribute to additional stress, thereby intensifying and perpetuating the problem.

When I worked in a correctional facility, I had an opportunity to observe dramatic, rapid weight gain influenced by stress. It was especially common among teenage girls. Norma is an example. When she arrived just prior to her eighteenth birthday, she was placed in a juvenile detention program. It was uncertain if she would be required to serve additional time in the adult women's prison after her birthday. As the time for the decision to be made drew nearer, Norma's anxiety level and her weight climbed at about an equal rate. She went from a normal weight to thirty percent overweight in a matter of weeks. This, in itself, does not conclusively prove a stress/obesity relationship. However, in the prison situation, where individuals' lives are so closely monitored, many of the variables that could have contributed to her weight gain but which could not be easily measured in a normal situation were observable under these circumstances. It was clear that stress was a direct cause of Norma's weight gain.

Norma was just one of a number of inmates, both male and female, that I was able to observe and monitor.

Individuals varied a great deal. Some of those under pressure would find it difficult to eat, experiencing the feeling that their stomachs were tied up in knots, and they lost weight. Others would eat a great deal more than normal under moderate pressure, but would lose their appetites when the stress increased. These same reactions were observed as a result of feelings of depression, loneliness, sorrow, joy, and excitement in other situations more commonly experienced by most people.

> **Stress and the resulting emotional/physical behaviors are a major, if not *THE* major, aspect of my holistic philosophy of weight gain/loss.**

In all my years of counseling, as well as my research with Schick's Shadel Hospital, I found that the stress/emotion factor that seemed to most often be the root cause of obesity was *FEAR.* Any time you perceive a threat to your person, your security, your desire, your needs, or your wants, you are apt to experience (as can be measured by biofeedback) some type of physical or emotional response that could be classified as stress. Great excitement, happiness, or joy can also be stressful. Your body does not distinguish between the types of emotions you are feeling, only the degree of intensity. Physical injury or illness produces stress, as does excessive fatigue, obesity, or the trauma of exerting vast resources of energy. In all these instances, your body (and mind) prepares to defend itself, balance itself, or flee.

WHEN *STRESS* BECOMES *DISTRESS*

Low levels of stress become distress if they continue over a long period of time. High levels of stress become distress rapidly. When stress becomes distress, it has progressed from a level that you and your body believe you can handle, to a level at which a breakdown, or even death, will result unless you get relief.

What is only mild stress for one person can be severe distress for another. It all depends upon how you perceive your own ability to cope with the particular situation or condition. For instance, a fifty-year-old man weakened from a recent heart attack is unlikely to believe he is, or could be, physically strong enough to handle as much physical or emotional stress as a healthy twenty-one year old.

A list of the causes of stress would be endless. All change perceived by your senses or imagined in your mind is stressful. Some stress experienced very early in life becomes a conditioned response. That is, you respond to just the *thought* of the stressful experience. Just thinking about a trip to the dentist, for example, is enough to increase the pulse rate and dampen the palms of many people. Some stress is very general, some is caused by very specific events, people, or ideas. Pollution, the economy, traffic congestion, war, rapid changes, crime, careers, unemployment, romance, your body image, drinking, smoking, poor diet, children, parents, friends, your philosophy of life, and your values are among the myriad potential sources of distress. What you believe about your environment and your ability to cope with it has everything to do with how you handle the stress or distress you experience.

The symptoms of excessive stress are almost as numerous as the causes. The following are some typical reactions to stress and/or distress:

* Illness — from allergies to cancer to high blood pressure
* Rapid pulse, heartbeat, or respiration
* Hysterical paralysis
* Muscle and structural problems
* Vision problems
* Inability to sleep or relax

* Tics or nervous gesticulations
* Speech impairments
* Loss of appetite or excess craving for food
* Excessive drinking
* Hyperactive behavior/excessive talking
* Disordered thinking
* Inability to enjoy entertainment
* Poor concentration
* Unduly serious/no sense of humor
* Little sexual satisfaction or impotence
* Loss of interest in old pleasures
* Short temper

STRESS MANAGEMENT

If you are one of those millions of people who are looking for more quality in your life by seeking a high level of wellness, you will realize that stress management is one requirement. *It is not necessary to wait until you experience stress symptoms to deal with stress.* Basic holistic health practices will enhance your effort to keep stress manageable and prevent distress. A quick review of these prevention practices is listed below:

1. **Self-Awareness:** an ability to sense what is happening in your mind and body in relationship to your environment. This is a natural ability which you can develop by simply practicing tuning in to yourself until it becomes a habit that is done without conscious effort.
2. **Exercise:** balanced, safe, daily, and progressive until you are in shape.
3. **Rest:** sufficient *restful* sleep/dreamwork and the development of waking calming routines and skills such as meditation, self-hypnosis, biofeedback, etc.

4. **Nutrition:** healthful eating routines, which eliminates sugar and salt; includes little or no animal fat; a variety of fresh fruits and vegetables; whole grain breads, nuts, seeds, beans; pure water in large amounts (1/3 more than you desire); no more than 45-60 grams of protein a day from yogurt, soy, nuts, whole grains, and sprouts; vitamin and mineral supplements, particularly vitamins B-complex, and C, niacin, calcium, and magnesium, in balance and moderation.

5. **Support system:** good contact with supportive friends and/or family.

6. **Calming activities:** pets, painting, expressive dancing, fishing, jogging, nature watching, gardening, etc.

7. **Environment:** air cleaners, negative ion generators; light — natural or full-spectrum; appropriate noise decibel levels; space — safe, roomy, some privacy; color — soft, natural, with bright colors as accents.

These basic factors are related to your stress levels and help to determine if other stress-producing factors will or won't become *distress*. These are also factors which you cannot always control completely. However, you can choose to give them a priority that will make them a part of your lifestyle so that when you are confronted with less healthful situations, you will be better able to cope.

If you are already starting to experience distress, the following steps will stop the escalation of your feelings and aid in reducing them to more manageable levels:

1. *Acknowledgement:* own your own feelings and be aware of them. Your ego can get in the way. Remember, bright people suffer stress also.

2. *Identify your emotions:* anger, fear, hurt, frustration, joy, peace, love, sexiness, hate, excitement. If you can

clearly identify the emotion you are feeling, you have more options for dealing with it.

3. *Identify the level of feeling:* is it slight and new? Is it strong and old? Is it a combination of many feelings at different levels? Are you just uncomfortable, or out of control? The sooner you identify the level of feeling, the easier it will be to deal with it.

4. *Ask yourself, "What am I doing with this emotion?":* are you building it up or down with mental messages? Are you ignoring it? Pushing it into subconscious storage for later use? Examining and dissipating it? Is logical behavior becoming illogical and self-defeating (overeating, drinking alcohol, smoking, violence, name calling, etc.)? The way you talk to yourself or project ideas with mental pictures will raise or lower the stress factor quickly.

5. *Express feelings positively:* verbalize — yell and shout how you feel, without attacking others or putting them down. Clarify — why and at what or who are you mad. Physically expend energy. Run, jump up and down, hit soft things that you can't hurt or that can't hurt you. Look in the mirror and act as upset as you can. Strain as hard as you can to *feel* as upset as possible. (Straining is a paradox.)

6. *Determine the true source of your stress:* Is it due to a conditioned response? Is it some fear you developed as the result of negative experiences long ago — and now you automatically respond to even the suggestion or thought of that negative experience recurring? Is it a new happening that you've worried about and predicted, and now it's being realized just the way you planned it? Is the source of stress coming from outside you (a friend was raped near your home), or something internal, such as gallstones? Is it a generalized discomfort you find hard to define, or a specific feeling? Does the stress come from a projection you are making into the future, a reflection into your past, or some-

thing in the present? Is it a primary (air, food, shelter) or a secondary (If I get a job, I'm afraid I won't be successful) fear? Is it fear of the unknown? What are the dynamics of your stress? Finding the source may require intellectual detective work, and just the *deductive process itself will reduce stress.* Finding the root cause or causes will offer more options for resolution of the stress by making your efforts more accurate and effective.

THE BASIC PRINCIPLES OF STRESS – COPING TECHNIQUES

All relaxation incorporates at least one, if not all, of the following seven basic principles:

1. ***Let down your defenses:*** Relax your muscles; quiet your mind; reduce the stimuli to your senses — sight, smell, taste, touch, hearing.

2. ***Have a focus point:*** One of your senses can be used for this by focusing on an object, a movement, a sound, a smell, or a taste. Your focus can be internal or external. It can be a mental picture of a flickering candle or a real flickering candle. The focus is on *one* single thing, such as your breathing.

3. ***Choose a safe place:*** It is important while relaxing not to be worrying about danger, interruption, or any type of distraction. Again, the environment should contain very little stimulus.

4. ***Start with an empty stomach and a fresh mind:*** It is best to practice relaxation on an empty stomach. If your stomach is active, it is more difficult for your mind to be calm. If you are tired and ready to fall asleep, you probably will!

5. ***Do not strain to relax:*** Straining to relax is a paradox. If you strain to fall asleep, you stay awake. If you strain to relax, you get up-tight.

6. ***Let go of the quest for magic:*** Almost anyone can learn a relaxation technique, but none of them are magic. To become useful, they require time, effort, energy, and sometimes they cost money.

7. ***Practice and develop a key:*** Each method, if practiced sufficiently, can be shortened in its process until just a thought, a word, or a mental picture is all that is needed to elicit the relaxation response. You will then be able to use the technique almost any time or any place, as needed.

So many of my clients want to be able to master relaxation techniques with little or no effort on their part, but remember, *the things you like yourself for, you must earn.* Quick and easy is for the movies. This is not to say that some people don't have a natural ability, and seem to do better and go faster than others; however, everybody who chooses to, can learn some relaxation technique if they make the necessary effort. If a client says to me, *"It* didn't work," they should have more accurately said, "I wouldn't open up to it," or "I wouldn't allow it to happen."

Some people want to relax but are afraid to, or they doubt their ability to relax. *Believing* you can learn to relax will improve your rate of success dramatically. You may fear relaxation because you feel you will become vulnerable or out of control. This happens to you if you believe your world is a very threatening place, and you don't dare take a chance.

The following techniques and methods are only some of the many that are available. Once you learn the principles, you can devise methods and variations of your own. Most of these relaxation methods are simple, do-it-yourself techniques. Some of the methods described may be best learned with a well-qualified instructor.

RELAXATION TECHNIQUES AND METHODS

Hot Tub — Bubble Bath — Hydrotherapy (Whirl-pool). Water seems to have a relaxing effect on many of us, especially if it is warm or moving. Watching water, listening to the sounds of waves on the shore, or riding in a boat that rocks you as your mother did in her arms can be very soothing.

Warm Milk and Honey. The sweetness and the warmth seem to soothe your stomach and relax you in the same way that a gentle warm hand massaging your stomach might. In the alcoholic ward of a Veteran's Hospital where I worked during my doctoral internship, we used this method instead of medication during the withdrawal period. While the effect was not as dramatic as drugs, it was sufficient to assist the patients through the difficult period, and they were often proud afterward that they made it through withdrawal without having to take drugs. Since these patients were already drug-dependent, this was an important accomplishment for them — a good way to start their recovery program.

Movement — Dance — Running — Yoga — Stretching — Martial Arts. Any one of these alone, or in combination, is excellent for reducing stress. I have practiced them myself for over twenty years. Your body holds emotional tensions locked into tight muscles, tendons, and ligaments, and when you move, you release that pent up energy, freeing yourself to be calm. Also, it changes your focus and thought process. Reading, classes, and/or private instruction are the best ways to begin.

Mindless Activities. Activities such as whittling or rubbing a worry stone require little or no thought, talent, or training, and serve no purpose other than to bring about relaxation, yet they provide a focus and movement.

Listening. Birds, wind chimes, music, and ocean sounds can be very relaxing when you focus *only* on the sounds. Even listening to another person talk can be a meditation, if done correctly. To relax, it is necessary to listen to the words with no judgements, analysis, or planning a response; only taking in the words and doing nothing with them in your mind. To listen in this manner is calming, and in addition, it helps you to hear in a way you usually do not — without any prejudgement.

Singing. Expressing your feelings vocally is a release, if done without inhibition. Singing, and music in general, can also elevate your feelings, depending on what kind of music you select.

Breathing. Different types of breathing can affect you in different ways. Books on breathing are available. Slow, deep, elongated, rhythmic breaths (without straining) are the most relaxing.

Art Work. Drawing, painting, sculpting, or working with wood, plastics, metals, or leather can be most tranquilizing. Working with your hands in an artistic pursuit provides a focus and a means of expressing feelings at the same time — without being dependent on words.

Juggling or Balancing. This practice requires intense concentration (focus). To stop for even an instant means dropping an object. These activities are, of course, not the deepest form of relaxation and serve for only short periods of time.

Massage — Hugs — Reflexology — Accupressure — Rolfing — Chiropractic — Napropathy — Shiatso. These are some healing procedures and/or tactile expressions that can be relaxing and generate positive, secure feelings. Some of these methods can be learned simply through reading. Others might require short courses, and still others years of professional career training. Hugs, of course, require no training — only sincerity. Both persons involved in this technique will be more relaxed.

Sexual Release. To be stimulated sexually to the point of climax is followed immediately by a deep sense of tension release. Biological cycles build a certain amount of sexual tension, which should be released regardless of what other kinds of stress factors may exist. If a loving partner is not available, fantasy along with masturbation is a normal, healthy process. Human sexuality is one area in which counseling with a professional may be helpful if fears, impotence or discomfort exist.

Fantasy — Imagery — Dreams. Mental pictures are a very big part of projecting and reflecting on thoughts that move your emotions up or down. They can stimulate you in any direction, and most people never learn to utilize them in productive ways that aid in dealing with stress and assist in reaching potentials. Your mind's mental pictures are a necessary part of creativity, motivation, dealing with fears and wish fulfillments and overall self-image. Learning how to direct and manage this element of yourself is a tremendous step toward self-responsibility, self-awareness, and self-actualization. Mental pictures are a powerful key to your emotions, and thus, your very meaning and purpose in life. Books, instructors, classes, and environments can all contribute to learning these skills, but I believe *practice* is mandatory to successful achievement.

Self-hypnosis — Autogenic Training — Auto Suggestion. These methods are very dependent upon mental pictures that are accompanied by your own verbal commentary. Using specific induction procedures and terminology, you guide yourself into altered states of consciousness — encouraging yourself to believe that you can do what you already are capable of anyway if only you did not doubt yourself so much. Again, reading, classes, and individual counseling with a professionally trained psychologist or psychiatrist can result in the greatest utilization of these skills. Listening to a record or tape which guides you can prove helpful, and individual attention will help assure your efforts are rewarded. Practice! Practice! Practice!

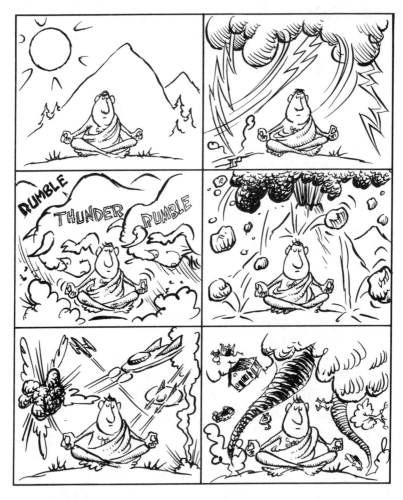

Meditation. This method differs from hypnosis, primarily in that you start by reducing the amount of mental activity down to a single focus. You concentrate on some object, movement, or sound that is without meaning in itself. While during the process of hypnosis you use a continual chain of chatter to yourself and imaging pictures to stimulate or relax yourself, with meditation you continue to focus on one thing. It is a narrowing down process. The focus is generally not associated with ideas that take you off into other areas of thought. Meditation and hypnosis both have unlimited induction techniques. A great many teachers are available on the subjects, as are organizations that use meditation as part of their core of beliefs. The depth of relaxation and the benefits from these techniques are also unlimited. One meditation method is described in detail in Chapter 18, "Putting It All Together."

Countdown. Closing your eyes, begin slowly counting down from one thousand to zero. Breathe deeply with each count, and imagine a relaxing scene in your mind. Concentrate on breathing in slowly and gently. This is an especially useful technique for falling asleep when you are tense.

Biofeedback. Simple home equipment that can be used effectively without professional training can be purchased for a very reasonable price. Using a meter, a light, or a sound, you are able to realize what level of tension you are experiencing at any given moment and in a continuum. Different instruments measure your muscle tension, your pulse, external skin temperature, or moisture emitted from your pores. As you receive feedback (signals) of the degree of tension you are experiencing, you gradually learn to sense how to mentally release or dissipate this tension. The process requires regular practice over a two-week period, and occasionally after that. This process can also be done without equipment by simply sitting with your hands in your lap, feeling your pulse, and concentrating on slowing it down. Also, it can be done by taping a small dime store thermometer to your wrist with the bulb touching the skin's surface, and concentrating on raising the temperature by increasing the flow of blood to the hand. Professionals who specialize in biofeedback can be found in most communities of any size, with much more elaborate and sophisticated equipment, that can measure several body functions at one time and provide printed readouts to more accurately measure progress. This equipment is more sensitive to smaller changes and is extremely useful in many ways other than just reducing general stress levels.

Progressive Muscle Relaxation. While comfortably seated, or in a prone position, close your eyes and think about your feet. Picture them in your mind's eye. At the same time, contract the muscles in your feet as tightly as you can for five seconds as you breathe slowly and deeply. Now, suddenly relax your feet as completely as possible. Next, focus on your calf muscles, repeating the concentration process, and then do the same with each muscle group right up to the top of your head. As you focus on each muscle group, concentrate on tightening only the set of muscles on which you are focused, and not the muscles around them. It is not necessary to stop breathing when you tighten a muscle group. Breathe easily, slowly, and deeply.

Implosive Therapy. Instead of *distracting* yourself from stressful feelings, encourage and expand on them. With imagery, attempt to exaggerate those things which upset you until they are totally unrealistic. Once you've imagined the worst, what you face in reality seems much less upsetting.

Paradoxical Intention. This is much the same as implosive therapy. In this case, you strain to be the opposite of what you want. For example, if you are angry and want to dissipate your anger, go to a mirror and attempt to feel as angry as you can. If you do this with a sincere, strained effort, you will probably start to laugh.

Bioenergetics. Screaming, yelling, hitting soft things, and acting out your feelings gets the stress energy out of your body. To get the most out of this exercise, work with a professional who is well trained in this modality.

Nutrition. The way you eat every day is very important in preventing distress and encouraging relaxation. High amounts of sugar, food colorings, caffeine, etc., can cause or contribute to stress, as can deficiencies of the B-vitamins, calcium, or magnesium. When you are under stress, certain vitamins, such as vitamin C, and minerals are used by the body more rapidly, especially if you drink alcohol or smoke. Some supplements, such as niacin or tryptophan can be especially helpful if taken in larger amounts than usual. Also, certain herb teas, such as comfrey or camomile, may be relaxing. As I mentioned before, it would be a wise idea to seek the professional advice of a nutritionist or nutritionally-oriented physician in planning the right supplementation for you.

Sensory Deprivation. This is a special technique, originally developed by Dr. John Lilly, **which should be used only under the supervision of a trained professional.** It is not useful for everyone, and could even increase stress for some people. The idea is to eliminate *all* stimuli. The patient or client floats nude in a saline solution of ideal temperature in total darkness, total silence, and total stillness for several hours. The effect can be very dramatic.

Restful Sleep. Because fatigue is a stress factor, restful sleep is one means of relaxation and coping with stress. Nutrition habits, anxieties, and dreams can determine how restful your sleep is. Sleep can also be used as a means of escape when the world appears too threatening *(psycho-asthemia)*. Drugs, smoking, and illness can interfere with sleep patterns as much as day-to-day worries. It is best not to eat within two hours of bedtime. The number of hours you sleep, and the time of day you sleep can be important factors. Learning a good relaxation technique to easily put yourself to sleep can be very helpful.

CONCLUSION

It should be remembered that stress, in and of itself, is a necessary part of life. You would probably not accomplish much or have little joy without it.

> **Whether *stress* becomes *distress* and results in blocking your potentials, limiting your efforts and joys, or resulting in illness or even death, is a matter of how you experience your world and your life and what you believe about your abilities to cope with stressful situations.**

When you live a balanced lifestyle and learn to believe in yourself, you can seek out change (stress) and feel even stronger for it. Your potential, when you are healthy (balanced) and relaxed, is unlimited. As a person, you become more attractive as your real self is seen, and life is exciting when your energy is not wasted in distress. In order to reduce inappropriate eating or urges to eat, stress management skills are essential. If you are wise, you will give learning and practicing these skills a very high priority in your life.

10

CHANGE IS WHAT COUNTS IN INCHES AND POUNDS

WHY DON'T WE LET GO?

Sandy (age twenty-four), Barbara (age thirty-six), and Donald (age thirty-two) are all members of the same weight-loss group. They seem to always have ten to thirty excess pounds they are trying to lose. They also continually talk about the changes they *should* make in their lifestyles and habits. They are all single, and each one feels that dropping some pounds and getting rid of extra inches would surely make a difference in their ability to attract an appropriate partner or mate. As important as this is to each of them, however, somehow the changes are very slow in coming or they are an on-again-off-again situation.

These three people are certainly not atypical. On the contrary, they are very typical of millions of other people who, for a multitude of reasons, wish to make similar changes that may result in lost pounds and decreased inches. Sandy has a frequent craving for Mexican food. Barbara has a tremendous need for candy every time she feels pressure at work and she keeps a supply hidden in her desk. Donald goes out with his buddies every Friday night to drink beer and chase women and ends his evening at 3:00 A.M. by having steak and eggs. The late night out minimizes the likelihood that he will feel like exercising on Saturday. All three of these people come back to group sessions each week with their guilt trips and confessions. Why don't permanent changes come about?

If we, as human beings, have the ability to carry out projected ideas and events (change), it does not seem logical that we should so often resist change by avoiding, denying, suppressing, and pretending — as if change were not inevitable, regardless of our unwillingness to deal with it. At other times *we may acknowledge that change is desirable, but struggle not to take any risks to achieve it; for example, many people replace sugar with an imitation sweetener.*

Change is more natural and inevitable than death and taxes. Even death and taxes are subject to change. Taxes keep going up, and death can often be either postponed or hastened by particular lifestyle practices. Change is everywhere and always. Everything is in motion, from the smallest subatomic particles to the cosmos itself. If Sandy, Barbara, and Donald look in a mirror and then at old photographs of themselves, or at their attitudes and goals of ten years earlier and their circumstances today, they can see that they are changing — and in some ways the changes are not at all what they want.

Some of these unwanted changes have been brought about by particular habits and lifestyle choices that have been established. Things we enjoy, even potentially harmful things such as smoking, can easily become habits. They become habits because we believe we enjoy them, and it is hard to change things we believe we enjoy. Change can be frightening because it is always an unknown, and unknowns tend to frighten us regardless of how well we are able to perceive things or how many reassuring guarantees we receive. If we don't like what may come next, can we return to what we had?

It may seem less risky to look for some kind of magic that will allow Sandy to have her Mexican food, Barbara her candy, and Donald his beer, steak, and eggs, and no exercise and still remain trim and shapely. But waiting for magic only seems to result in even more extra pounds and inches. The circle of bad habits, extra pounds, and guilt feelings goes round and round and the only change that takes place is that the pattern increases in intensity.

Resisting change is like trying to push back the river, so why not go *with* the river ("go with the flow"), or even get out in front of it and direct it — make it work for you.

> **The real question is not how to avoid or resist change, but how to direct it.**

Continuing with Sandy, Barbara, and Donald, the self-improvement changes required to achieve their goals seem readily apparent: Nancy simply gives up Mexican food, Barbara gives up candy, and Donald gives up beer and extra meals. If, however, we look a little more deeply, we begin to see why it may not be quite so simple. We discover that Sandy has not developed any supportive friendships and spends too much time alone, which intensifies her compulsion for Mexican food. Barbara feels that her job skills are weak; thus, she feels an exaggerated sense of pressure which increases her dependence on the sensual comfort of candy. Donald is afraid to approach women that appeal to him, so the night out with "the boys" seems important, contrarily, both as an avoidance of facing women and as a vain hope that he might be braver with his buddies close by.

In the cases of these three people, not only is giving up the inappropriate eating habit necessary, but also changes must be made in their way of relating to others.

The first step toward self-improving change is identifying accurately the changes to be made. This requires looking a little deeper than the surface problems. Sandy, Barbara, and Donald are involved in group counseling, which is an excellent place to begin exploring changes, but a formal group isn't mandatory. Friends and people who know you well can often be helpful in this process. Sometimes it is hard to let down your defenses sufficiently to look at yourself objectively, and supportive friends can help you feel safe enough to recognize desirable changes.

The second step toward change is being *ready* for change. Making changes wisely, with consistency, requires time, attention, prioritizing, sometimes a financial commitment, inconvenience, and also courage to face fears. An important indication of readiness is when you quit looking for something magic, or for some other person to change the circumstances, and begin looking into yourself for internal change.

> **Readiness is *wanting* to change, not just feeling that you *should* change. *Should* is for other people; *wanting* is for you! After you know *what* you want to change and that you are *ready* to change, it is time to examine *how* to change.**

Important personal changes that you are committed to are changes that are self-initiated. It is important not to feel pushed or forced. Using freedom to act on your own behalf leads to greater effort, greater desire, greater satisfaction, greater belief in yourself, and additional positive changes because the person doing the changing (you) is the person receiving the credit for the success and effort. Self-initiated changes can be made on your own terms, which is very important to the next step.

The third step toward change is relaxing and letting down defenses. This means that your mind and eyes are open to see and understand new possible ways in which to change. Opening your vision is necessary to imagination, intuitiveness, innovation, and creativity. It is also necessary in order to see objectively when you are falling short. As your awareness of expanded options increases, greater relaxation is experienced. Expanded thinking, awareness, and relaxation go together and can all contribute to the process of making positive personal changes.

Because you may tend not to feel safe at first, it is helpful to begin with small changes. Make small changes in a process of building up to ultimate big changes. It is usually easier to assure success with small changes, and this success helps you gain confidence to make bigger changes. You may even want to make some small changes unrelated to weight loss just to get started. *It is important to focus on the idea that you are becoming a **self-directed** changer.*

Often I will suggest that people get started by practicing using their non-dominant hand to do a particular chore or chores that have been done in the past with the dominant hand only, continuing these practices until they become ambidextrous at certain tasks. This helps keep the focus on change, it builds confidence, and the challenge can be fun.

Trying to be rigid in making changes is like the mighty oak in the wind. Rigidity creates tension and uses energy that can bring fatigue, which may lead to a break. *By taking a rigid (obsessive-compulsive) position, you find little joy in your effort to change and you will tire of it soon rather than learning to prefer the change.*

Taking the opposite position — blowing like a leaf in the wind — is also defeating to positive change. The leaf goes wherever the wind blows it; no direction or purpose is established. If you try every possibility for change that comes along and don't stick with any one thing for very long, little self-growth will be realized. Obviously, some middle point is desirable.

It is a good idea to stick with a change long enough to determine whether it is an improvement or not, while remaining open to other possibilities. Once a certain change is accepted as useful, it is still possible to remain open to new and even better possibilities while continuing to be consistent about the most recent change.

LETTING GO

> **Change is often more a matter of relaxing and *letting go* than forcing or struggling to make yourself different.**

When you find it hard to concentrate, to be consistent, to deal with emotions, or face a fear, it is like the struggle to change — the desired change may come about easily if you simply quit struggling and let go. Let go emotionally so that you can let go physically. It doesn't matter what you are letting go of — the process remains the same. When you let go and the struggle is over, you have changed to the point where you are now comfortable with what used to be a problem.

Donna had been on her weight-loss diet for three months and had lost the same seven pounds twice. She desperately wanted to lose her extra forty pounds and she knew what she had to do to lose it, but she could not be consistent in her efforts. She would go along for a few days, or sometimes even for a week or two, being very strong. She would follow all the tips given to her in her weight-loss club, do her exercises faithfully, and then, suddenly she would find herself confronted with an offer of fresh donuts at coffee time, or stopped in front of the ice cream section at the grocery store. She was like a marathon runner who hits the imaginary wall twenty miles into the race. The emotional urge to eat ice cream or donuts again was so strong that she could almost taste their sugary softness melting in her mouth as she fantasized about them. Her logical self kept reminding her of her commitment to losing weight and how well she had been doing. However, even if she were able to pass up the donuts or ice cream this time, once the mental conflict began, it never seemed to stop. This struggle with herself would go on until she finally gave in and broke her diet, which, of course, would result in guilt, hopelessness, and more donuts and ice cream.

This scenario is played out in the lives of millions of people every day in response to innumerable desires. Emotionally, the person wants something, usually something they have had many times before — something with which they have had many pleasant, satisfying associations. It could even be something they have only had many wonderful dreams or fantasies about. Now, however, the logical mind has been convinced that it would be beneficial to give up that special something (for example donuts and ice cream). There is a *desire* to change or to "let go" of the inappropriate object of affection, but the struggle seems to go on. The conflict in the mind is between what is *desired emotionally* and what is *believed logically.*

This situation is painful and energy draining. Why does it continue for so long? Like the dry alcoholic who struggles for years not to drink — isn't it just a matter of time until his energy runs out, his resistance breaks, and he takes the next drink, with relief that the struggle is finally over? Why does the struggle go on at all? The very struggling *not* to have something, *not* to do something, or *not* to eat something, seems to almost guarantee that if the struggle doesn't end, eventually the result will be inappropriate behavior. The struggle is fatiguing. The more we struggle, the more it wears us down. Pure will power seldom works.

But what keeps the struggle going? Let's talk about Donna again. She did a number of things to keep her struggle alive:

* She kept her focus on what she was trying to give up.
* She doubted her ability to get along without it or replace it with something equally satisfactory.

* She shut out other, maybe better, possibilities for the future.
* She felt her security was in what she had known and was comfortable with.
* She kept a continuing analysis going about her struggle — verbally with others and silently to herself.
* She reinforced the fear that she was giving up a reward, as if it could not be acquired again in new forms.
* She stayed within contact, sight, sound, and smell of the very things which she was struggling to give up.

HOW CAN YOU LET GO OF THE STRUGGLE BEFORE YOU BREAK?

Donna was distracted from her struggle when she took up meditation and applied it to her walking exercise. It made the walking so much more refreshing and enjoyable that she began walking much longer distances. She was amazed at how far she could walk and how rapidly she could cover the distance. This was a success and gave her a feeling of self-control which she then used to project an image of herself jogging in 10K runs. She began to believe she could train to jog 6.2 miles, and as she realized her focus had changed, she went in a new direction. *The struggle was over.* Her goal now was not to lose weight, but to get herself in condition to jog 6.2 miles. She had changed her focus from a negative desire (not to eat inappropriately) to a positive desire (to get her body in shape for the 6.2 miles).

How to let go was never really a clear issue with Donna. She came upon it accidently when she opened up briefly during meditation and realized the joy of movement and its possibilities, which helped her realize that she could change. She learned to believe more in herself as she used her freedom to take action that brought about lasting change.

People use:
    distraction
    substitution
    organized behavior modification
    belief (faith)
    intellectual awareness
    self-development
    mental and physical exercise
    support groups
    opening up to a new focus
and many other active efforts to let go of the fight before it does them in. The struggle itself becomes a means to let go (change).

THE PROCESS OF LETTING GO

The actual process of "letting go" is very difficult to describe. A physical description of muscle relaxation is analogous and particularly suitable because of the familiar image of muscles relaxing. You've experienced muscle relaxation, and it is part of what happens when you let go emotionally. Once you have let go emotionally, the graphic description of the process is relatively unimportant, as you realize it is primarily a sensing process.

If you think back on the experiences in your life when you did let go emotionally of something that had been very important to you, you may remember what it *felt* like when you let go even if you didn't analyze *how* you were able to let go.

Another technique that can be useful in letting go is implosion. With this method, you not only stop avoiding what you are afraid of and start examining it, but also your fear is taken into fantasy and exaggerated and blown up by embellishment to the worst possible end imaginable. Once you have dealt with the worst possible experience in your mind, the possibility of a less exaggerated experience happening in real life loses its threat.

The following example illustrates this process. Recently a young woman came to me expressing a fear of saying "no" to other people. She was continually finding herself out on dates she didn't want to be on, working for committees whose causes she didn't believe in, and eating foods that her mother and friends pushed on her. Her fear was that if she said no, she would no longer be loved, accepted, or respected. During several sessions, I asked her to imagine herself saying no in various situations, fantasizing the worst possible result; seeing herself being rejected, put down, and left alone. I told her to stay with those images until she could see herself recovering by her own social skills. Then she could go on to practice saying no in ways that would not offend other people. After she had mentally faced the worst and survived, gradually bringing "no" into her daily vocabulary was not nearly so threatening.

> **"Letting go" is always easier when you are headed for something you want and when you believe you have already faced the worst, even if it is only in your mind (which is usually the only place the "worst" really exists).**

Reflecting on the many changes that have already come about in your life, you will quickly realize that most changes are neither fatal nor final. The changes keep coming. *The question is how many of the changes will you control?* Given all the limitations you have on your choices to change, you still have tremendous freedom to move around within those limitations. As a rule, people do appear to be much happier, more fulfilled, and healthier when they direct their own life changes, and I think you will be too.

11

FEELING FREE

THE EXCITEMENT IN HUMANISTIC EXISTENTIAL BELIEVING

Commonly, when we are feeling depressed or incapable of dealing with life, the obstacles, questions, and challenges seem to "make" us feel locked in and controlled by circumstances — certainly anything but free. The feeling of freedom to many of us is the idea of having no financial, physical, social (ethical-moral), environmental, or occupational restraints upon us.

This idea of feeling controlled or locked in is common with my overweight clients. To hear a client blame his spouse, children, parents, culture, heritage, emotions, or some other "unchangeable" circumstance comes to be expected. It is easy to have empathy for the conditions and pressures they share with me, as I have felt many of these same pressures myself. In the past, as these stories of seemingly insoluble plight were being told, I felt a great deal of pressure to *rescue* the client; to somehow save him — to free up each person from the limitations the world had put on him, which had resulted in his body and mind falling victim to unending obesity.

In stepping back from the intensity of each moving life narration and viewing all the stories in a larger philosophical context, I began to see the confines we have all felt as something we were *locking ourselves* into. We are often our own jailers. To verify my observation, I set up an experimental group of twelve people, each with the commonality of being more than twenty percent above their ideal weight. The group met for two hours one evening a week for a period of six months. During this period, I never weighed,

97

measured, or used any supportive or therapeutic technique other than the group itself. Diets, exercise, or weight loss were never a focus of discussion. The discussions were limited to a presentation by the clients of encumbering life circumstances: people; events; personal, emotional, physical, and psychological experiences. As the group members gave their reasons for being forced to continue on a self-defeating path, I would play devil's advocate and confront them with alternatives. The choices, at first, were denied and put down as being impossible, unrealistic, or foolish. I, myself, frequently saw the courses of action as being difficult, costly in time, energy and money, or frightening and inconvenient, but I always asked the question, "Do these alternatives present true options?" With the passing of a few months, the group members began to acknowledge that, although the alternatives which I presented were not anything they would seriously consider doing and that these alternatives presented consequences they were not prepared to live with, the choices truly *were* options. As time passed, the options were more readily accepted as being difficult or frightening, but not necessarily impossible. It was also at this time that noticeable weight loss was becoming apparent. As group members became more and more able to accept the idea that they always did have choices, we discussed their new, broader, more flexible views of themselves as *free*, with the potential to become the people they wanted to be. By the final session, each person had a clear understanding that in a significant way he determined the quality of his own life, the manner in which he experienced his world, the development of his emotions and even the pounds on his body.

The following is a typical example of a group discussion about choices:

Mrs. D.:   "I have no choice about feeding my teenage children a certain amount of junk food, or they won't eat at all."

Dr. McClernan: "What would happen if you only prepared quality food?"

Mrs. D.: "They wouldn't eat at all, or they would
only eat junk food after school and get
sick."

Dr. McClernan: "Does that mean you don't have a
choice?"

Mrs. D.: "Well, I would feel terribly guilty as a
mother if they didn't eat, or if they
became ill."

Dr. McClernan: "Does that mean that you don't have a
choice?"

Mrs. D.: "My husband, parents, and kids would
all be angry with me or would think I
was crazy."

Dr. McClernan: "Does any of this stop you from refus-
ing to buy junk food or serve it with
meals, or does it really mean that it
would be a difficult choice which may
cause you some temporary complaints
or upset?"

With many exchanges of this kind, the prison doors began to open.

This existential group did as well as other groups I have conducted which utilized self-hypnosis, aversion conditioning, nutritional counseling, etc. Fifty percent were still maintaining their ideal weight after one and a half years, which is excellent in the world of weight loss.

If your personal philosophy of life includes the belief that you are always free to make decisions that will influence your life, and that choices are always available, the value structure by which you live will place your awareness of options high and you can find many more directions to go. This is just what the growing, self-adjusting person needs in order to reach unlimited potentials.

To some people, the ideas here may sound selfish —
reminiscent of the "me" generation of the sixties; however,
there is a difference between the enhancement of the "self"
and being "selfish." When you learn to be self-adjusting,
your life will go more smoothly, you are more relaxed; you
are able to reach out to others more, be more understanding, be more able to love. Everybody you contact benefits by
your growth. This self-enhanced person, then, is not selfish.
This is a humanistic-existential decision-making person who
models for others and moves more comfortably about in the
world of change.

HUMANISM

When we hear the term "humanistic," we usually think of
an individual or group being sensitive in some way to the
human condition: understanding, accepting, empathizing,
allowing for human weakness, faults, mistakes, etc. Humanism may well include these traits, but I'd like to put it in more
positive and comprehensive terms by offering a definition
formulated by the Association for Humanistic Psychology,
an organization of which I am proud to have been a member
since 1966, and for which I have actively worked for several
years. A humanistic person:

1. Centers on experiencing as primary to understanding himself and others.
2. Affirms his or her fundamental uniqueness and the
   importance of human life.
3. Tries to develop, enlarge, and expand the human
   experience.
4. Believes that intention and values are crucial to
   human choice.
5. Emphasizes attention to self-realization, spontaneity, loving, choosing, creativity, valuing,
   responsibility, authenticity, transcending, and
   courage.

6. Seeks means to integrate the whole person — emotions, intellect, body and soul.
7. Is concerned with the individual, the exceptional and the unpredictable, rather than only with the regular, the universal, and the conforming.
8. Explores synergistic relationships within groups, communities, and institutions.
9. Has fundamental commitment to a total view of the human experience.

EXISTENTIALISM AND FREEDOM

It would be extremely difficult for any person who accepts, believes, and lives out the above definition of humanism to deny the existential philosophy of life. In my view of the human condition, we who are able to think and decide are existentialists at least at a minimal level — even if our only choice is to lie down and do nothing more until we die, it is still a choice.

> **Existentialism in its briefest definition would be simply *THE QUESTION*, the ambiguous, subjective question continually faced every conscious moment.**

Should you read the next line? Should you believe what you read? Should you scratch your itch? Are you alive? Is there a God? Everything of which you are aware becomes a question, including the question, "are you aware?" If you decide you are aware, then you can decide what you are aware of, and you can choose to become still more aware. If you become aware of choices, you realize you are free to make a decision. As you continue through life, experiencing and changing is constant. Thus, the opportunity to make choices is almost unlimited. This type of existential awareness frightens many of us, because it is saying that within limits, for example, physical restraints (I can't jump off the Earth), we are responsible for who and what we are. It is easy to think of a situation wherein choices are difficult and limited, but you are still free. An example is Victor Frankl's German concentration camp experience, where lines of naked Jews were being marched at gun point into crematories. Even in this horrible, seemingly hopeless situation, Frankl realized he had choices. If nothing else, he could choose how he would die. He could run and be shot quickly, wait and hope something would save him, drop to his knees and beg, cry, laugh, scream, refuse to move, or even find meaning in his own dying. When you accept this existential truth, you also stop seeking magic.

Accepting the idea that you can never escape your existential decision making may seem like a lonely, uncertain, frightening thing. However, **if viewed positively, the existential choice is also your freedom.** Freedom to think your own thoughts, to feel your own emotions, to act out your own behavior. People or circumstances may make your choices either easy or difficult; however, you can still choose and commit yourself to becoming self-actualizing, thereby creating meaning and purpose in your life. Life can be an adventure instead of a horrifying nightmare. You can even transcend yourself on occasion, as did Neal Armstrong when he stepped on the moon for mankind. If you choose only to accept your own values, you can free yourself from tremendous guilt and use the energy that went into guilt for new pleasures and self-directed changes.

You not only determine your own values, but you also determine your own rewards. If you take a humanistic existential position and attitude, your rewards will be as unlimited as your choices. You'll always have clear, self-fulfilling directions. You won't be either rigid or a leaf in the wind, but rather balanced, flexible — a determinant of change. Problems, challenges, and needs become opportunities for your own growth.

Briefly, the existential process is summed up as follows:

* **Awareness** — the more aware you are, the more options you have.
* **Choice and Decision** — you are free to choose to be more aware.
* **Responsibility** — you may also decide to accept your new responsibility for yourself.
* **Commitment** — you are free to decide to commit yourself to the decision-making process.
* **Experiencing/Change** — experiencing and change are continuous with the above factors, providing unlimited options
* **Self-actualization** *(becoming the better self)* or **Transcending** — because you have the options of all of the above factors, you are able to seek your potentials.

No special sequence of the steps in this process is necessary for the realization of your own freedom.

On one level, all of us who think and decide are existentalists. On another level, no person ever fully completes the process. By its very nature it is unending and never perfect, yet meaning in your life comes from your effort in the existential process. To repeat, existentialism most simply defined is, then, "the question." The ambiguous, subjective question you face every continuous conscious moment you live.

> **You've been free since you started making decisions. *What will you do with your freedom?***

To accept the humanistic existential concept for yourself will assure success in your efforts to deal with your weight and to go on to a self-actualizing lifestyle. These ideas about being free are centuries old. I have only attempted to apply them to a special situation — the desire to lose weight — and offer them to you who truly desire expanding the possibilities of your own life.

12

BEHAVIORAL PSYCHOLOGY AND WEIGHT LOSS

It is my opinion and belief that the two schools of psychological thought, *behaviorism and humanistic existentialism,* are never completely separated; therefore, as a holistic practitioner, I attempt to utilize both, and not to struggle with which one is better or more effective.

Speaking from a non-technical point of view, behaviorism is a system of rewards or punishments used to condition behavior—to reinforce positive, self-improving, learned behavior, and to discourage negative or self-defeating behavior. Supposedly, we all set up patterns of functioning based on stimuli (cues), rewards, and fears, which condition us to act as we do — simple cause and effect. Theoretically, it should, therefore, be unnecessary to go deeply into psychoanalysis to improve a situation. We must simply change the system (patterns of stimulus) until we are reconditioned to the more desired responses.

This is all very acceptable to me as an existential humanist, **if** the subjects being conditioned are fully *aware* of the conditioning process going on and are taking part by their own free choice. This last sentence will make the pure behaviorists curl up and die, as they do not accept the concept of free choice as a possibility. But as you can see by the central theme of this book, I believe that *we can be* aware, and *we do* make choices, even though we do have physical-intellectual limitations with environmental pressures that make our choices either easy or difficult.

One weight-loss organization which employs aversion conditioning (faradic shock) indicates that the subconscious mind is conditioned in the same way Pavlov's dogs were. Using biofeedback, it has been demonstrated that the human subconscious mind is a better discriminator than the conscious mind; that people do not condition in the same way as rats and pigeons do. People who think of themselves as intelligent often feel that it is demeaning to submit to being electrically shocked for eating a hang-up food. In my research, I did find, however, that even though the subconscious mind was not conditioned to believe that each time a treated person approached a hang-up food an aversion would take place, other benefits were derived. Some people saw the shocks as a symbol of their commitment to change. Other people found it easier to accept the idea that existential change to better ways of eating was a personal decision. Still others claimed that they felt they actually *were* conditioned (at least psychologically — maybe even by suggestion) and experienced nausea or imagined pain prior to taking a food for which they had been conditioned to have an aversion. I am not against the use of aversion conditioning, as long as people using it have awareness of the aversion conditioning process and as long as they know they are freely choosing to use it — because then it is not seen as magic.

If you wish to take a more formal, detailed approach to behavior modification, you can make it extremely elaborate and, if necessary, employ a professional behaviorist to assist you. Behavioral techniques can be very effective, and I am in favor of their use, *as long as you know what you are choosing, how the techniques work, and that you are making use of the techniques on your own initiative.* If you believe it will work and you realize the energy to make it work is yours alone, I'm sure you will benefit from it.

To take a more structured approach on your own, you might start by keeping an hour-by-hour account of patterns of your behavior over a two-week period. Many people are overconfident that they are already aware of their behavior, and thus would not benefit from keeping the journal, however, most people who do keep a good, detailed log of their daily activity are surprised at how much they learn about themselves. In your log, list what you are thinking, feeling, and what is happening around you at the time you are engaging in a particular activity. In a couple of weeks, you should be able to determine your conditioned habits and the cues to those habits so you can begin to set up your rewards and/or punishments on a new schedule. If you are consistent in following your plan, in time the new behavior will become a habit — and then you will prefer it. Here's an example: You might learn from your journal that you automatically have a snack every afternoon at 3:00 P.M. in front of the TV set. In fact, maybe you learn that you snack every time you watch *any* of your favorite TV shows. So, in an attempt to change your behavior, you rearrange some of your viewing schedule. For example, maybe instead of the 3:00 P.M. soap opera, you may watch the early morning exercise show (give yourself a non-food reward). Maybe you even make a rule for yourself that food can only be eaten in the kitchen, at meal times, and that if you do anything while watching TV, it must be some type of exercise (as long as you don't see it as punishment). If you go through all of your habits, you can set up a whole program of new behaviors with appropriate rewards.

Rewards have proven to be more effective than punishment. In my own research, I have found very few people who are willing to punish themselves. However, no matter which you use, you may want to consider having a relative, friend, or professional help you with this project. This person should be someone you trust to be consistent, interested in you, serious about what you are doing, and someone who will not try to take matters into his own hands to do more or less than you requested. Accept your freedom/responsibility to choose, and success will follow.

TRY A CONTINGENCY CONTRACT

A helpmate hands out the rewards or punishments which *you* decide to use. Use the rewards or punishments to change habits of eating, exercise, reading, relaxation practices, group participation, and social development. Rewards can be anything you value, except food that is unhealthy or in quantities that are too large. Money is often used. For example, you could give your helpmate a large enough amount of your money so that it is very important to you. Then, draw up a written contract outlining all of the contingencies you must meet to earn the money back. Each contingency is given a progressive or final value. That is, if you fail to meet a particular contingency one time, it will cost you, say, $5.00; the second time, $10.00; and the third time, $20.00 — or, if you wish, the total amount you've invested. Some items you may want to assign such great importance to that if you break contingency requirements even once, you lose the full investment. To keep your helpmate honest and objective, any money lost should go to the charity of your choice. (See the sample contingency contract in the Appendix.)

Provisions should be written into the contract to cover such things as illness or other reasonable emergencies. One clause should cover your pleading to end the contract before the agreed-upon length of time. That is, if you attempt to get your helpmate to change the agreement, you lose money.

> **This is an honor system, and if you think, know, or feel that you can or will cheat on the contract and be able to look your helpmate in the eye and lie, then don't even bother to attempt it.**

The contract can cover as many contingencies as you like, but more than ten becomes difficult to keep track of. If the volume of change is overwhelming, a negative attitude may result.

HOW THE CONTINGENCY CONTRACT WORKS

The following case of Thelma is a good example of how the contingency contract can work. Thelma was a 45-year-old woman with a serious heart condition, who weighed seventy-five pounds more than her doctor recommended when she met a man a few years older than herself and fell in love. In recent years she had been very depressed and lonely. She was divorced, and her children were grown, independent, and had moved far away. She had considered suicide several times. Her lifestyle *was in itself* a slow form of suicide. Now, however, she was highly motivated to change as she wanted very much to be with this new man in her life.

Thelma was only seven years old when her mother had died at a young age. Thelma had very strong memories of being close to her mother and sitting on her lap and eating candy. Even to this day, the warm, happy, safe, and loving memories came back whenever she would eat candy. With such a strong association between candy and a loving, safe environment and relationship, this compulsive habit would not be easy to break. Thelma agreed to undergo psychotherapy, coupled with a holistic program using a behavioral contingency contract. She put five-hundred dollars into her contingency fund, which represented a sacrifice in terms of her income and expenses. She requested that this money be turned over to the Heart Fund in part, or completely, if she did not live up to all or parts of the contingencies she specified — lowered food intake, specific types of food to be eaten or avoided, exercise, and meditation practice.

For almost two weeks Thelma did well; then suddenly she appeared at my office unexpectedly. She was in tears and very angry and frightened at the same time. She wanted to end the contract and forget the whole thing. She was especially angry with me for suggesting the idea, and was certain she couldn't continue for another eight weeks, although she had made it this far without a slip-up.

After two hours of talking, relaxation techniques, and positive reinforcement, Thelma agreed to proceed, day-by-day, to the end of the ten week period. The crisis was over, and each time I saw her after that she was much improved. She began to develop faith in her ability to change, and by the end of the ten weeks, her new belief in herself, coupled with the thirty-pound weight loss, was enough to bolster her the rest of the way to a new lifestyle, renewed health, and increased feelings of well-being. She still fantasized about those moments with her mother, but it was brought about by her own ability to use imagery and focus on the relationship itself, not the candy. Her new love relationship and her new image of herself took away much of her need to live in the past.

In this example, existential decision, a humanistic relationship, psychotherapy, and a behavioral technique were put together, *by Thelma,* to bring about more than she had imagined possible in her life. She realized in retrospect that the change may have come about even without her new love relationship, simply because she made the decision that she wanted to change.

USING PUNISHMENT

Usually self-administered punishments are pleasures you deprive yourself of, according to how much and how frequently you fail. In some commercial programs, faradic shock or drugs to make a person vomit are used. These techniques should not be used without the aid of a professional. Another punishment to avoid without professional guidance is the sensory deprivation room or tank, where you are placed in a space for a period of time, with no sensory input — no sound, no light, no tactile sensation, no movement. This could be dangerous without the guidance of a competent professional. In fact, I suggest you stay away from any physical punishment in a self-help program.

Depending upon how it is viewed, exercise can be seen as either a reward or punishment. For example, it can be offered as a reward break from reading your nutrition book, or as a punishment for eating a piece of cake. However, since you want to introduce exercise into your permanent lifestyle and become addicted to it, thinking of exercise in terms of a reward is more apt to be beneficial.

IMAGERY

Another potentially powerful tool that is, to me, both a behavioral and an existential technique, is imagery. In your mind's eye, you see most of what you think. You fantasize pleasant things and experience pleasure. You fantasize unpleasant things and experience fear or discomfort. If you imagine taking a big bite of a freshly cut lemon, your throat contracts or you salivate. Imagery can be used to reward and punish yourself. An example would be to see yourself slim, running easily and rapidly on a sunny beach, as a reward for having a vegetable salad for lunch. On the other hand, as you reach for a cupcake, visualize yourself bulging out of your clothes as you're puffing and missing your bus because you can't run. You use your mind's eye every day, and by dreaming at night, you act out your feelings. Why not deliberately make this imagery work for you? Learning to use imagery is also helpful in other self-development techniques discussed in other chapters.

In this chapter, I have given you basics upon which to build by personalizing them to your own needs and circumstances. A plan is not completely set up for you. It will take your own initiative, energy, decisions, and effort to put it into use. Now you know about it, so you have a choice.

(A more complete guide for those who wish to incorporate behavioral psychology into their programs is an excellent book by Joyce D. Nash, Ph.D, and Linda H. Ormiston, Ph.D., *Taking Charge of Your Weight and Well-Being*, Bull Publishing Company, Palo Alto, CA.)

13

GETTING FAMILY AND FRIENDS ON YOUR TEAM

Given the world in which we live, efforts at changing routines, habits, and patterns of living can be very difficult. The influences from your environment can be so strong that, at times, it may seem as though attempting to resist the many pressures *not* to change is like swimming upstream. Access to food and reasons not to exercise seem to be everywhere and always.

Because you spend such a large percentage of your life either at home or at work, family, friends, and associates are able to have a tremendous impact on your behavior, thinking, and feelings. The well-intentioned people in your life who care about you most, are also the most able to sabotage your efforts at changing. Even though these important people want to help you, their very caring for you, their misperceptions of what you really want, or their own wants and desires blind them to the negative effects they can have on you. If their own lives are out of balance, it makes it still harder for them to see you clearly, to get outside of themselves and to be useful to your cause.

Certain people in your life may find the fact that you want to change threatening, as *your* changes may be seen as bringing about changes in *their* lives or their relationship with you. As long as you stay the same, they may feel secure with you. Change, on the other hand, is an unknown, and that can be threatening — if they are not prepared for it. Other people in your life may welcome your changes and feel, in fact, that change is long overdue. These people may be over-zealous in their eagerness to help and put over-whelming pressure on you.

Ann was a person who had set herself up to be chief cook and all-around-maid even though she had worked outside the home most of her married life. Her husband and college-age daughters had come to take her for granted. When she started a weight-loss program which included classes, exercise routines, support group meetings, and the purchase of new and different types of food, her family became noticeably upset. They did not mind if she lost weight, but they did not want her to stop waiting on them and to start making changes in *their* eating habits. It would mean each family member would have to do much more for themselves, and they would not have the food they had become accustomed to unless they purchased and prepared it themselves. Their reactions, not surprisingly, were very non-supportive and uncompromising. When Ann's husband and two daughters recoiled from her changes, Ann felt over-whelmed, and immediately returned to the old way of life, feeling hopeless and resentful, and afraid to try again.

Marsha, a high school senior, seemed to gain pounds in direct ratio to her divorced mother's degree of distress with her work, lack of adult relationships, and being a single parent. Most of Marsha's friends had similar kinds of stress in their lives and seemed unable to lend real support to her efforts to lose weight. Marsha retreated to her room and TV as the stress became greater. She did not know how to seek or build a support system, and it's likely that her problems would have become worse if her mother hadn't sought professional help for herself. Of course, as Marsha's mother's distress improved, so did Marsha's weight problem.

Those with whom you live, play, eat, work, etc., on a daily basis have a tremendous influence upon you. Some-times, where weight loss is concerned, it is negative; other times it is positive, and commonly it is a combination of both, as with Marsha and her mother.

From my observations, I have found that those attempting weight loss who prepare their families and friends in an organized, consistent manner do the best. When people know what to expect from you, they feel safer; even if they do not care for all of your changes. If they are asked to participate, most of them will at least feel appreciation for being asked, and everyone will know where the other person stands and what obstacles will need to be worked around.

ORGANIZE A TEAM

One method of assessing the cooperation and support that can be recruited is to approach family and friends as though you were organizing a team — a team that can be of benefit to all its members as well as those who choose to be spectators. However, those who join your team should profit the most.

To form a support team, start by paying close attention to all of the people with whom you interact regularly. Notice what each person is doing with his or her own exercise and dietary habits. Pay attention to their attitudes, values, and moods. Check to see how they are interacting with you and what roles you have with each other. Some of these people are probably assisting you in your subconscious effort to stay overweight. However, *they* are not responsible for you as an individual. The question is, when you do find something negative in your relationship with another person, how do you change it to something positive?

Although a mediocre team effort is more helpful than no effort at all, you only want those people who truly want to be on your team and who are willing to work toward the goals you and the other team members agree upon. After you have taken the time to make your observations you might want to gather all of the possible team members together to make your mutual decision about joining the team. Sometimes this is done best by having a party — a "getting skinny" party.

Plan your party to have much physical activity of games and lively dancing, followed by low-calorie, healthy munchies and drinks. Preceding the snacks, you may even want to hold a group meditation session. As the activities proceed, notice how involved the people get. How willing are they to try, and how much do they complain or express satisfaction?

After the meditation, start your discussion session by explaining your goals and your desire to form a support team that hopefully will benefit all who take part and bring each of you closer together. Even though *your* concern may be weight, each person may have a different concern or goal. Let each one state his or her own concerns. The essence of your team activity is to be supportive in whatever manner you can when your paths cross. A team can be as few as two people, or as many as eight or ten.

Some people may want to leave you at this point. If so, let them go easily. Avoid asking them to just give it a try. What you are really looking for is a commitment — an eager person who sees value in the concept for himself. Where very young children are involved, it can be viewed as a game with rules, and you may be surprised how much they enjoy it, while reminding you of your own commitment. For those who still want to leave at this point, wish them well and ask them at least for a commitment not to interfere with the team. If anyone leaves with hard feelings, let them know you care about them and how they feel, but that your resolve remains strong. Get together with them privately later, if possible, when they have had more time to accept your decision.

With those who elect to be a part of the team, initiate the following discussions (beginning with yourself) by offering your open, honest opinions, intentions, and commitments. Be prepared to hear and accept some things that don't feel good.

1. Discuss openly with each person how you feel about fat, fat people, and especially your fat and their fat, or lack of it.
2. Discuss with them your weak points in exercising, eating, relaxing, and so on, and their behavior that influences you positively and negatively.
3. Discuss ways in which you might help them achieve their goals.

Each person should talk to every other person, individually, using tactfulness, but remaining open and honest. If you have something to say that the other person may be sensitive about, before you bring it up, qualify your remarks with the positive feelings you have for that person, and let him know of your fear in bringing the matter up — you don't want to lose his friendship or cooperation. Tell him something like "this is hard for me to say, as I'm afraid you may reject me and I care very much about remaining friends; however, I'm going to trust that you will understand, so I'll take a chance."

Each person may not get exactly what he wants (some may want more than others); therefore, compromise and social adjustments may be necessary. Ask that all requests be reasonable and feasible, and not attempts to pass individual responsibility on to others.

Get down to the nitty-gritty. You may want to draw up a written contract. Even though the contract isn't legally binding, it can carry ethical obligations and help avoid future arguments. Another good idea would be to plan regular brief meetings to make adjustments to your original plans and to assure that as many needs as possible are being met.

Support groups can be the single most important factor in losing weight and keeping it off. If those people with whom you live and associate are unable to provide good support for you and each other, an outside group is even more important. Before giving up on the home group, make sure you've given it an honest effort. You may want to go so far as to hire a professional for one organizational session or to help with adjustments after the group is underway.

> **The most important point for each person is that you *don't depend on someone else!* Give 100 percent, hope you get 50 percent in return, and figure anything you get back is a bonus.**

The number of people living alone has grown tremendously in recent years, and those attempting to lose weight who are living alone may need a support team as much or more than those living within a family unit. Although the single person is better able to control his home environment and activities, with fewer people to consider, there also may be other potential difficulties with which he has to deal. Loneliness and inappropriate eating frequently go together. When the support team is concentrated in the home, it becomes of much greater importance. Friends and associates at work, school, clubs, church, etc. should be cultivated. Special interests and causes also serve in a support role, as they can give meaning to life.

To the single person, romantic interests and sexual relations (or the lack of them) can greatly enhance or detract from the weight-loss effort. The close sharing, sensitiveness, and communication of a romantic involvement can be very helpful if there is clear understanding and appreciation of your goal. The partner may have an equally difficult task, which allows for mutual sharing of support and modeling. Relationships where only one partner, or neither partner, is attempting positive self-development, put greater strain on any weight-loss effort and reduce the chances for success. The single person needs the team support, and staying in contact with the team (in a balance with being alone) will increase the strength of the weight-loss effort.

14

HELP SOMEONE ELSE WIN THE BATTLE OF THE BULGE

If you truly want to help someone you care about lose weight, this chapter is written especially for you. You can play an extremely important role, even if the overweight person is not seeking your assistance. On the other hand, without a clear understanding of the overweight person's needs, your good intentions can influence the addition of pounds.

The overweight person in our contemporary, weight-critical society is apt to be emotionally sensitive and full of self-doubt and guilt regarding his extra pounds. If this person has been chronically overweight, it is likely he will have clear feelings of inadequacy. This means that even sincere, well-meaning questions can be heard as hurtful attacks or put-downs. No matter how cheerfully or calmly the overweight person may seem to accept your remarks, it is no assurance that damage has not been done. This does not mean that open, useful discussion can't be developed over time; however, it is most effective when nurtured in proportion to the rate at which the person attempting to lose weight is finding success.

Overweight people are no different from anyone else. We all tend to be sensitive about what we see in ourselves as weaknesses. As we begin to overcome our perceived short-comings, we are also much more open to discussion and even confrontation. If approached at the right time, in a non-aggressive, sincere, well-meaning manner, even the most sensitive overweight person can be confronted to his benefit.

TALK TO HIM ABOUT HIS WEIGHT

Readiness for discussion is indicated when the overweight person not only has had some degree of success through his own efforts, but also when he initiates a discussion about his weight. Serving as a stimulus, you can start a discussion about your struggle with your own weaknesses — whatever they might be, about the overweight person's strengths, or about neutral subjects. Ask sincere questions. A sincere question should be delivered in a noncritical tone of voice and should not imply an answer. Any questions about which you are not sincere build distrust. Your relationship with the overweight person is a good subject with which to begin your discussions. The time, place, and atmosphere to start trust-building discussions is most important. You should both be relaxed and free from distractions, and the meeting should be in private.

CONFRONT HIM ABOUT HIS WEIGHT

"Helping" and "stimulating" can be two very different concepts. *The Oxford American Dictionary* defines *help* as follows: "To do part of another person's work for him, or to make it easier for a person to do something." To *stimulate* means, however, that by acting as a stimulus, you rouse a person to activity.

Confronting a person before he is ready will only bring up his defenses, or encourage rebellion or withdrawal. Confronting can serve as a stimulus only at the point when the overweight person feels safe with you and he has had some success. In order for him to feel safe with you, you must not only be open to being confronted yourself (without being defensive), but you must also nurture the overweight person's confrontation of you regarding your own weaknesses.

REMEMBER, HE'S IN CHARGE

At the start of the overweight person's efforts, keep your suggestions to yourself. Even if you are asked for help or advice, stick to questions (i.e., "What would you like to do?" "What will that mean to you?" "What are your choices?", etc.) If you are asked to monitor an activity or administer a reward or punishment, do so only by following his directions. If you feel that you cannot be consistent or that you will be patronizing, don't accept the job. It is extremely important that the overweight person knows he is making his own choices and that he can take credit for any success. Whatever you do with him at his request, cooperate only if he is doing the work. It is best if he is able to reciprocate by performing a like service with you — a true trade-off.

EMPATHY IS IMPORTANT

Know that weight problems are not simple problems, with a single cause or cure. Weight affects all aspects of the person's life, his view of himself and his world. He is involved in an internal conflict, and the struggle can be just as strong whether he has ten pounds or two-hundred pounds to lose.

The experience of being overweight can be painful, handicapping, and frightening. It results in the loss of self-confidence, self-worth, and self-esteem. Feelings of guilt, embarrassment, shame, frustration, and anger are common; just because an overweight person jokes or laughs about his size does not mean these feelings don't exist.

Most overweight people have been victimized by more than one false promise of a magic cure for their condition. Thus, they may feel vulnerable and abused, possibly depressed, or even hopeless and helpless. It is very hard to empathize with these feelings unless you recognize a struggle of your own that is equally hard.

ARE YOU ACTUALLY ENCOURAGING HIM TO STAY FAT?

One thing a person close to the overweight person frequently overlooks is his own possible interest in keeping that person overweight. It has been my experience many times in my work that when the overweight person started to change, his spouse or another family member has become upset to the point where they have phoned me, come to see me, or even threatened me. One reason I've initiated family orientation in my program is so that important people in the overweight person's life will be prepared for changes and will be able to make adjustments of their own.

When the overweight person begins to make changes, these changes are rarely restricted to weight alone. The person may become more assertive, change his habits around the house, become more social outside the home, go back to school, or go to work full time. All of these changes can be potential threats to family and friends. The person is no longer predictable, and the unknown can be frightening. As the overweight person gains self-confidence, many previously hidden desires may come to the surface. If a woman begins to lose weight, her small children may think, "Mom might leave us." Teenagers can think, "She won't clean our rooms anymore, or do our laundry and make meals, or be at home whenever we need her." A husband might think, "More men will be attracted to her, and she'll be out in the world where they can take her away from me." Or worse yet, the husband may think, "I'll lose 'control' of her. As long as she is overweight, she needs me."

As a friend or family member, you need to remember:

1. By losing weight, the overweight person will become healthier, and that will add to your relationship.

2. He will be happier and more fulfilled, which will inevitably add to *your* life.
3. He will be more appealing to you physically.
4. You shouldn't want to keep this person a prisoner of his weight or feel responsible if the excess weight causes health problems.
5. This is an opportunity for you to improve your life too.

HELP SOMEONE ELSE BY HELPING YOURSELF

If you really think about it, helping an overweight person is an opportunity to build your own ego or self-image. We usually get a lot of good feelings — of worth, importance, sharing and being needed — when we know we are helping. If you take a position of arrogance or superiority, even if you think you are helping, you are actually causing harm by bringing out the other person's defenses. Whenever you can't understand why he can't simply use willpower, you are not helping, accepting, or even seeing yourself very clearly. I've yet to meet a person who has not, at some time, given in to his feelings instead of following logic. Overweight people often overwhelm themselves with their feelings. The idea is to balance logic with emotion.

THE ROLE OF THE SUPPORT MEMBER OF THE TEAM

What is needed from the thin support members of the team is that they be close by as models or examples. *Not models of being thin, but rather models of being honest, open, accepting, and understanding people who are in self-development struggles of their own — people who are being consistent and successful in going through their own painful growth.* Examine your own needs, attitudes, values, habits, skills, fears, and body with some objectivity and with input from the overweight person, and I'm sure you'll find some things about yourself equally as hard to change as being overweight.

In setting up your own developmental program with an overweight person, you become a primary support person. It is very important to be honest, consistent, accepting, committed, and open, and to avoid lecturing, nagging, and teaching the virtues of your rightness. You can offer your feelings about your own struggles and express your sincere belief in the overweight person's reaching his goal. If your help is not sought out, you can still serve best by entering your own development program, and asking for *his* support, saying nothing about the overweight person's own program. It is *crucial* that you be sincere about your own developmental efforts. If you are not — or if you are inconsistent and give up on your announced commitment — you do more harm than good.

When you are being a good model by getting into your own development, you are truly sharing. One thing you need to share is support. You can be cheerleaders for each other by applauding one another's successes. How and when you applaud is important. First, praise must never be offered unless it is sincere. Second, it is best to applaud in proportion to the success. If it is a small success, you will come off as phony if you make a major production out of it. It may be good to save up several small successes before giving praise. Approval is worth more if it is given intermittently and moderately until major hurdles are surmounted. Your applause should be given more intensely at the start, and should diminish in frequency as development continues, but should increase again as the final goals are in sight.

Your general attitude and belief about the overweight person is extremely important. If you really do believe he is going to make it this time, his chances increase. People frequently live up to the expectations of others.

> **An overweight person is responsible for himself and is free to make his own decisions. That you cannot be responsible *FOR* him, but rather *TO* him, is important.**

If you want to be responsible to him, you must consistently (not rigidly) keep your own act together. Even if he wants you to be responsible for him, you *cannot*. We all experience our own emotions, think our own thoughts, and act out our own behavior, and nobody else can do it for us. This awareness is your freedom to be who you want to be. When you accept the responsibility to determine who and what you are, it gives you cause to like yourself. Don't cheat the overweight person by trying to assume his responsibility. It is his chance to like himself and to realize his freedom.

Unlike the view held by some clubs for fat people, the overweight person is a whole that is made up of parts, and each part affects the others. A fat person is not just an overweight person. He is an intellectual person, a sexual person, a spiritual person, a social person. He plays many roles at work, home, and school — parent, child, spouse, and friend. If your focus is on what he can become, rather than simply on the loss of fat, his chance for permanent change increases. When he is developing all aspects of his life and his goal is to like who he is, the fat will disappear.

One of the most important things you can do is to listen. How you listen is very important. Practice listening without judgement, analysis, or preparing a response. When you listen in this manner, you will hear as you never did before. Simply take in the words and do nothing with them until the speaker is finished. When you do this, you aren't ready to respond when the speaker is done. Only after the speaker is finished should you formulate a response. Most of the time all you need to do is to hear and accept. You don't have to agree, as long as he knows you heard him and accepted him as a person with feelings and ideas of his own.

Of course, there are the obvious practical steps you can take:

1. Don't treat the overweight person as handicapped; assure him that he can do things for himself.
2. Eat a healthy diet yourself.
3. *Invite,* don't challenge or nag, the overweight person to exercise with you.
4. Let go of snacking!
5. Keep conversation positive; don't go to either extreme of avoiding or focusing on the subject of fat.
6. Read self-help books.
7. Learn to calm yourself.
8. If fat bothers you in any way, let him know, but don't dwell on it, criticize, or put him down for it.
9. Continue to let him know you care about him.
10. Share your concerns about yourself and ask for his support.

Your greatest help to the overweight person in your life is simply to work on becoming the best person you can be for you.

15

LOVE RELATIONSHIPS CAN BE WEIGHTY PROBLEMS

The connections between what appear to be love relationships and weight problems are many and varied. In this chapter we will examine a few extreme examples, realizing that your situation may be significantly less involved, but at the same time you may identify some similar issues in your own life. The idea is not that a love relationship by itself is ever the single cause of weight problems, but rather a possible contributing factor that is often overlooked.

ROMANCE

Joan had been raised by critical parents who helped her believe that she was good only for household chores, and to feel she must be dependent on a man for her very survival. By marrying at an early age, she went from child-dependent to wife-dependent, and she was quickly divorced by a suffocated husband. Suffering from feelings of failure, inadequacy, and guilt, she did not want to return to the home of her critical parents. Instead she went through a long series of brief relationships with men. A few times she felt that she was deeply in love, but each romance ended unhappily, and Joan was left feeling rejected and unworthy of love. After each painful "love" relationship ended, she would turn to the only sensual comfort she could count on — food.

As she grew from chubby into obese, the only relationships with men that Joan seemed able to establish were with older, father types, or very dependent people, such as herself. The relationships continued to end in the same old way, with Joan feeling worse about herself each time, eating more, putting on additional pounds, and believing her search for "Mr. Right" was even more hopeless. The quest for a love relationship was finally ended when she quit seeking the perfect relationship and focused on building a meaningful life, a career, and a support system of friends and activities which developed a belief in her own ability to maintain a healthy body. A healthy love relationship soon followed.

HUSBAND-WIFE RELATIONSHIP

Jane and Ray are two former counter-culture people who have become part of the establishment. Ray is now a successful corporate lawyer, and Jane is a housewife and mother in the most fashionable part of suburban Phoenix. Even though they both maintain many counter-culture views, they now do so in a quiet way. They are careful not to rock the comfortable material/status boat they live in.

During the sixties, when they lived the drop-out, rebellious, casual lifestyle, both Jane and Ray had chidren out of wedlock with other partners. Having both come from traditional middle-class backgrounds, they felt tremendous insecurities when they became single parents. Jane and Ray still feel alienated from almost everyone — from their own parents, the counter-culture group, neighborhood groups, and professional associates. They only feel comfortable with each other.

Jane is at least seventy pounds overweight, and food is clearly an important part of the communication between her and Ray. She has the power in their relationship, and Ray does not dare challenge that or express any feelings that are not positive. They each feel they are deeply in love with the other and will not do anything to threaten these feelings.

Only because Jane's health is being jeopardized by her excess weight are they considering counseling.

During counseling, Jane and Ray displayed their intelligence with rationalization that was both insightful and clever. While both acknowledged their fear of losing the other, neither dealt with those insecurities. They seemed to believe that if they destroyed their mutual dependency, the security of their life, as they now knew it, would also be destroyed. They were in a very difficult situation because of Jane's health. As they saw it, if Jane lost the weight, they would risk losing their love relationship. By not facing their fears and making some changes, Jane would stay fat, and her health was in danger.

PARENT-CHILD RELATIONSHIP

By her senior year of high school, Penny's parents had been divorced for six years. Although her father's business was close by, Penny did not get to see him often due to his busy schedule and his new girlfriend. Penny was most distressed by her father's leaving, and her security was clearly threatened. Her mother, a nurse, was angry and hurt by the divorce, and was left feeling very insecure and inadequate as a woman. She seemed to feel more comfort and support from her older daughters, which left Penny, who had been closest to her father, even more alone.

Feeling deserted, anxious, and with no one to turn to, Penny reached out to the sensual comfort of food. When she had gained forty extra pounds, she realized she had finally found a way to get attention from both her parents, even though it was in the form of criticism. She withdrew from school friends and activities and developed a series of psychosomatic problems which resulted in several extended hospitalizations and lots of attention.

As a high school senior, with her older sisters gone from home, her mother seeking new relationships, and having to face the prospect of leaving home for college herself, Penny was torn between losing the limited love relationships she had, and getting herself together enough to establish new, hopefully healthier, relationships in the near future. With the support of counseling (along with her mother), and a weight-control group, she began to let go of the manipulative behavior which she had been using to get attention (love) and re-established her relationship with her peers. Being bright, Penny had been able to *understand intellectually* what needed to be done, but *emotionally* she found it painful and difficult to make the changes until she began to realize that healthy love relationships offered a great deal more than just having attention directed at her.

Although these three case examples are all different, they have several similarities:

* The overweight person is using the comfort of food as a substitute for an incomplete or unsatisfactory love relationship.
* The weight serves as a false sense of security.
* The weight brings new problems or conflicts.
* The weight is intermixed with other aspects of their lives in a way that the weight problem improves or worsens in direct ratio to the "love" relationship or feelings of insecurity.

IS IT LOVE?

It is questionable whether love relationships that are built upon dependency, insecurity, fear, and manipulation are healthy love relationships, or even love relationships at all — they may be only strong feelings of dependency, inadequacy, and insecurity that are relieved with a mis-perceived sense of being loved.

It is true, as has so often been said, that "we must love ourselves before we are able to love others." When you are very caught up in your own emotional needs, it is doubtful that you will be able to extend love, because your focus and energy goes into your own need to survive. Then too, society tends to teach us to make ourselves lovable rather than learning to love. As a male, I've been lead to believe that if I achieve power and status, I will be assured of love. Women are assured love by their beauty, sexuality, or weakness (many men need someone to dominate).

If you are too involved in your emotions to love yourself or to extend love to others, or if you are too busy trying to make yourself lovable to learn how to love, you can easily mistake your insecure feelings of wanting to be safe and loved as your love for another. Chronically overweight people can easily find themselves in this position and misidentify their emotional fears as feelings of love. No matter if the excess pounds were there prior to the love relationship, or if they came after, when you seek out a dependent relationship, it is often a sign of feelings of inadequacy. If you have strong feelings of inadequacy, chances are good that you will be attracted to someone who shares these feelings of inadequacy, even though your behavior and personalities may appear to be quite different. In the initial attraction, mutual needs make for acceptance and empathy. In the long run, however, these unmet dependency needs lead to resentment, greater and new fears, and self defeating behavior, such as inappropriate eating. The lonely, single overweight person can so easily fall into this trap.

Other reasons why obesity gets people confused in *love-need* relationships and why walls are set up against the development of a *love-fulfilling* relationship become more and more obvious. For example, Jane, a wife and mother, is praised continuously for the especially tasty (but fattening) meals she prepares. Gradually, she begins to perceive her worth (the reason to love her) as her ability to provide delicious food for her family. She believes that if she were ever to change her role of fat cook, her family might not love her anymore. She tried to change to a more healthy style of cooking once, but all the fussing and complaining frightened her and further reinforced her belief that the main reason her family loved her was because of her cooking. So, she slipped back into her old role, which keeps her in the kitchen overweight, dependent, and scared. Is this love?

THE OVERWEIGHT PERSON'S DEADLIEST LOVE

Food and drink, sensual as they are, can be a medium or stimulant for sexual involvement. Making love and gastronomical pleasure can easily become an extension of one another. This association can even be carried to the point of saying that refusal to either take or give sensual food/drink pleasure is to say, "I don't love you anymore." The development of this situation can be so gradual and subtle that it may never be recognized either by the people involved or outsiders. The excitement of touching each other can gradually shift to the excitement of shared taste delights. Food and drink can be symbolic to the love relationship, or the focus of it. In either case, weight problems are apt to ensue.

The love relationship that can develop with food itself is apt to be the most unhealthy and hardest to change. If you fall into this relationship, you may view food as a dear friend, a non-verbal confidant that always understands you and accepts you in a non-critical way. Food is also able to give sensual highs. It can look beautiful, with wonderful textures and colors. It can be warm or cool. It can be easily found and brought along with you. It doesn't care how attractive you are, if you're rich or poor, young or old. No matter who you are or how you look, it can be yours. It's easy to see how a love for food can develop and how it can be hard to give up when there are no prospects for other fulfilling love relationships.

Even when the feelings for food have degenerated to a love/hate relationship, which almost always happens, the conflict and struggles are understandable. Once you are involved with food so completely, its negative aspects are revealed. However, it isn't just the excess weight, with all its social, psychological, health, and occupational price tags, it is the realization that the positives felt for food were also negatives. Food may not be such a good friend after all. It isn't a confidant, because it tells everyone who sees you what you have been doing and feeling. It doesn't always accept you in non-critical ways. It can come back at you in a variety of physical discomforts, health problems, or even death. It will let you make a fool of yourself. It may make you feel high at one moment, and depressed and guilty the next. It can feel and look awful as a symbol of tremendous trouble and pain. It is everywhere, and seems impossible to escape. It can be the very devil in disguise — a taunting lover with no understanding or forgiveness, that laughs, mocks, and ridicules when you fall for it. Like any addiction, it evokes desire and hatred at the same time. Paralleling a close relationship between two human beings, all the elements for the negative and positive are present. Food can be a wonderful source of life-giving sustenance, or a silent killer. But one thing it will never do is *take the place* of a healthy love relationship between two people.

Whether you want to enhance an existing relationship or begin a healthy relationship, the procedure is the same. You must focus on your own development. To become a good partner, a clear sense of self-identity and worth is required; a self-initiated confrontation with personal fears, seeking out your individual potentials, establishing balance and flexibility in your lifestyle, and a habit of searching for your better self in body, mind, and spirit. These efforts lead to inner security which is what gives you the ability to reach out and love. It gives you the ability to go beyond just needing and manipulating to being self-aware enough to know when you are in a position of strength. Then you can establish a strong, healthy, flowing love exchange that nurtures itself and remains in good contact with the larger world and your own being.

DEALING WITH THE CHANGES

In my weight programs with growth groups, individual counseling, behavioral self-management, relaxation training, etc., I have found that it is common for participants not only to lose weight, but also to become more assertive, expand their activities, start or further a career, go back to school, request more variety and frequency in sex, change food purchasing habits and pay more attention to personal grooming. With all these changes, the mate is apt to become confused, angry, or threatened.

I suggest at the very beginning that the overweight person bring his family in for orientation to help prepare them for changes that may occur, to help familiarize them with program goals, and to elicit their support. The support that is requested of the family is seldom what they expect. I don't simply request that the mate or family change their diet or administer rewards or punishments for good or bad behavior, or that they serve as cheerleaders or monitors (spies), but rather to embark on their *own* self-development programs. (See Chapter 14)

We strive to establish a sharing partnership where each person serves as a model by working on his or her own potentials. If only one person in the relationship is self-actualizing, the chances of their growing apart increase. When both partners make positive changes, they reinforce one another and both become more able to *give* love, not just to *need* love. The couple or family becomes accustomed to change, which is what life and love relationships are all about. When all are growing as individuals and unreal expectations of each other are diminished, losing weight is just a part of the success that is achieved.

ESSENTIAL ELEMENTS OF A HEALTHY LOVE RELATIONSHIP

All potential love relationships, be it between singles, married couples, parents and children, or friends, require the same components to be healthy and love-fulfilling:

* **Good communication** — clear, honest, frequent, and open!
* **Realistic expectations** — own your responsibility for your own happiness, success, and liking who you are; don't expect perfection in others.
* **Value priorities** — each of you lives up to as many of your own values as possible and respects the other person's right to hold different priorities.
* **Healthy lifestyle routines** — in a flexible manner, practice exercise, good nutrition, and relaxation techniques to keep your bodies and minds in good shape and in a state of development.
* **Resolution of personal fears** — identify and face your fears on your own initiative, in a gradual, but persistent way that doesn't overwhelm you, instead of avoiding and hiding from them.
* **Building a strong support system** — nurturing meaningful involvements with friends, activities, causes, and beliefs, so that you are not dependent on one person and you can bring real additions to your love relationships.
* **Fair fights** — instead of struggling for dominance. No violence or verbal put-downs.

* **Sharing** — instead of mutual dependencies and control.
* **Self-actualizing modeling** — instead of criticism and jealousy.
* **Balanced/centered life** — instead of extremes of anything.

A truly healthy love relationship does not nurture obesity, and healthy love relationships come only to those who are healthy in themselves.

16

WHAT *IS* THE RIGHT DIET?

"Perhaps nothing in the world arouses more false hopes than
the first four hours on a diet." — Dan Bennett

A person who has learned to listen to his body has
become sensitive to hearing the subtle, and sometimes not so
subtle, messages it gives. When these natural sensitivity skills
are combined with some basic knowledge of nutrition and a
commitment to label reading, weight-loss diets, as such,
become worthless and a frivolous waste of time, energy,
money, and health.

This chapter defines the common basic weight-loss diets,
describes how they function, and denotes some problems
with them. It continues by discussing general nutrition for
good health (which includes a natural-sized body); how to
become your own best judge of your ever-changing nutritional needs; and how to learn to prefer the food that keeps
you functioning at your best.

A quick stop at your local bookstore will probably
uncover more than three dozen "surefire" diets *guaranteed*
to make you lose weight fast, effortlessly, and enjoyably.
Each diet book is written by a doctor or health specialist with
impeccable credentials (or sometimes no credentials at all),
and the cover strains to convince you that true magic has at
last been discovered.

Let's look at some of these diets critically in an attempt to
evaluate their various approaches to weight loss and to
separate dietary fact from fiction.

First, remember that if you follow any of these diets, losing some weight is absolutely no problem. The matter is, not however, solely a question of losing weight; the question is what quality of weight will you lose, and will you be able to keep it off after completing the weight-loss diet?

There are three basic sources in your body for weight loss: **water, protein,** and **fat.** If the weight lost is mostly water (achieved by following a diuretic-type diet, one of the commonly-used reducing diets), the weight is regained very rapidly once you return to normal eating patterns. This necessitates a return to the diet to lose the same (water) weight over again, and back and forth. We all know people — you may be among them — who are on and off diets repeatedly. This is not an effective means of weight control.

Protein makes up the muscle mass of your body, and an ill-conceived diet can cause you to lose weight from the protein of muscle mass, leaving you weighing less, but in a muscle-compromised state, at the end of your diet. Specialists in weight loss talk about *lean body mass,* which is a measure of the weight of your skeleton and muscle, and they use this as an indication of how effective a weight-loss program has been. The minimum percentage of the body which should be made up of muscle and bone in fit individuals is eighty-five percent for males, and eighty percent for females. This means that if you are an acceptably fit male, fifteen percent of your total body weight can be fat, and if you are a female, twenty percent of your body can be fat. On a good weight-loss program, the percentage of body fat should decrease as you lose weight, thus demonstrating that the weight you are losing is coming from fat, thereby improving your fitness — not coming from muscle, the loss of which would decrease your fitness (even though it is also decreasing your weight) over the long term. To accomplish this proper weight loss (fat loss) exercise combined with reduced food intake is the answer. *More exercise — less food.*

> **The most effective diet program is one that causes loss of *fat*, and encourages you, once you have achieved your desired weight, to maintain proper body weight and lean body mass through a prudent and nutritious diet, without need for continued weight-loss dieting.**

A LOOK AT THE COMMON DIETS

Let's take a look at the five basic dietary weight-loss programs commonly used today, and examine what influence each of these diets has on your body. The diets are called by many different names, but all of them can be classified into one of these five categories:

1. *Low-calorie mixed diet* of about 1,000 calories a day.
2. *Monotonous low-calorie diet* of about 500 calories a day.
3. *Ketogenic diet* of high fat, high protein, low carbohydrate.
4. *Starvation diet*, using a fasting procedure.
5. *Modified protein-sparing / partial-fasting diet* of about 300 to 500 calories.

Each of these dietary regimes will encourage weight loss, some resulting in a faster loss than others. Some people report that they can lose fourteen or fifteen pounds a week on a particular diet, and hail it as the "only way to go." An inspection of this amount of weight loss, reveals that much of it has come from water and muscle protein. How do we know that? Each time you lose a pound of fat, your body must burn it up as energy from the store of fat in various cells called *adipocyte* cells. To burn up a pound of fat requires approximately 3,500-4,000 calories of expended energy. Putting it another way, you would need to jog approximately thirty miles at an eight-minutes-per-mile pace to burn up a pound of fat. Therefore, if you lose fifteen pounds in one week and it all comes from fat, you would have to expend 60,000 calories for the week, or more than 8,000 per day, which would be impossible unless you are a logger, cross-country skier, or in training for the Pittsburgh Steeler's upcoming season. The average person who is dieting expends no more than 2,000 calories a day in activity. Therefore, it is impossible to lose that many pounds from fat alone. The majority of the weight will have to come from water and muscle protein loss.

Why muscle protein? Because muscle protein, when used as energy, contains less than half the stored energy potential per gram as does fat tissue. Therefore, *you can burn off muscle two and one-half times faster than fat with the identical calorie reduction.* It can be seen, then, that some diets may lead to fairly substantial weight loss in the early stage of the diet, but it most likely will be producing only extensive water loss and compromising muscle mass, which was hard won in the first place.

There are modifications and variations of all the basic dietary approaches. However, let's examine the five basic types in detail.

1. **The low-calorie mixed diet,** which uses reduced amounts of food from the various food groups, is without question, the safest diet and the one that shocks your body least. It is, however, the most difficult for many people to stick to, and the one that leads to the slowest rate of weight loss — generally one or two pounds a week. For people hoping for quick answers to difficult problems, this dietary approach is not satisfactory, even though the rate of weight loss, as well as the diet itself, is the safest and most desirable.

2. *The monotonous low-calorie diet* uses single foods or groups of foods in large amounts (such as grapefruit, eggs, apples, or any other food of low-calorie content). Eating enough of any one food ultimately kills the appetite, simply because you get sick of seeing that food at every meal. This is a very nice trick, then, to encourage you to lose your appetite and thus to lower your food consumption considerably. However, people do get disenchanted with the same food or group of foods day in and day out, and soon lose interest in this diet.

3. The so-called *ketogenic diet,* which eliminates all carbohydrates and recommends high protein and/or fat consumption, is often hailed as the best weight-loss diet. Some of these diets suggest that you don't need to regulate the quantity of your food intake at all as long as you eat only protein and fat. A simple examination of the dynamics of weight loss points out the ridiculousness of this statement. The amount of weight that you lose *has* to be tied to the difference between the number of calories that you are expending each day and the number of calories that you take in each day. If you are taking in large amounts of calories in protein and fat and maintain the same activity level, then you will *not* lose fat weight as fast as if you cut down on the consumption of calories. It is, therefore, impossible to lose fat from your body, no matter what foods you eat, without cutting down on calorie intake.

The ketogenic diet, a classic example of the diuretic-type diet, will produce weight loss, most assuredly, but that weight loss comes predominantly from water. The high-fat, high-protein diet produces a considerable amount of water loss, because it increases the blood level of a byproduct of fat metabolism called *ketones.* Ketones are produced by the body in response to a high-fat dietary intake. In fact, any time you reduce food intake, the breakdown of your own stored fat will produce some ketones. The difference then, between a normal diet and a ketogenic diet is that the ketogenic diet, which includes larger amounts of fat, will encourage more extensive ketone production. Ketones accumulate in the blood and produce the effect of increasing its "saltiness." As the blood becomes full of ketones, and subsequently more salty, it will tend to draw water out of the cells of the body to try to dilute the salt, and this water ultimately passes out as urine, thereby resulting in a diuretic effect and weight loss. But, this weight loss does not come from the desired stores of body fat, and lean body mass shows virtually no improvement during the course of this type of diet.

The ketogenic diet produces one other highly undesirable side effect. Ketones are also acid in nature. An increase in ketones increases the acid content of the blood, producing a state known as *ketoacidosis*. Ketoacidosis can be quite dangerous for certain sensitive individuals. It can cause changes in the contraction of muscles such as the heart, and have toxic effects on various organs throughout the body, including the liver, kidneys, and brain. If the ketone content rises too high, coma and even death can result. Most individuals can avoid ketoacidosis by drinking more liquids to flush the ketones out of the body and by taking supplements to replace the minerals, such as potassium, which may be lost. The bottom line however is that this diet will not significantly improve lean body mass, it does have some potential adverse side effects, and therefore it should not be used by anyone who is truly concerned about improving his level of fitness, developing proper food selection habits, and maintaining his weight after the diet is broken.

4. **A starvation (fasting)** diet uses diluted juices as the only food source. While it is clear that starvation has to cause weight loss, it is also clear that it is not the best way to achieve weight loss. First of all, in the beginning two or three days of the starvation diet, most of the weight loss comes from

muscle mass. You must stay on a starvation diet for approximately three to four days before your body will begin to use fat as its main fuel source to keep the engine running.

> **The starvation diet also depresses the thyroid and actually *lowers the basal metabolic rate*, which is somewhat like the idle speed of an engine. As the idle speed is turned down, your body consumes fewer calories while resting, and *you actually decrease the rate at which weight can be lost.***

The starvation diet, or fasting dietary approach, like the ketogenic diet, results in increased ketone levels. If ketones are not monitored carefully and appropriate fluid intake encouraged, ketoacidosis can develop. Much of the euphoric state that seems to be associated with starvation or fasting is apparently caused by ketone buildup in the brain and a subsequent biochemical response of the brain to the ketones, which is felt as mood elevation or altered states of perception. It is not uncommon for people who have been fasting for some time to have to be forced off the fast because they feel so good. They have arrived at a state of "karmic" consciousness during the fast as a result of anesthesia of the brain produced by the toxic buildup of certain metabolites. Although the individual may feel euphoric, the diet could have been having some detrimental biochemical effects.

A check of urinary ketones, using "keto-sticks" which can be bought at your local drugstore, will allow you to assess the buildup of ketones in your body. You should not register a ketone level of more than "2 +" during the course of your diet. If it becomes higher than this, you are developing potentially toxic levels of ketones and balanced nutrition should be reintroduced.

5. The last general dietary approach is the **protein-sparing/partial-fasting diet,** which, theoretically at least, sounds as though it is the best approach. Variations of the protein-sparing diet are all designed to accomplish the same end: that is, the body will lose weight almost exclusively from fat, without wasting or burning up muscle. The way to do this is with dietary replacement of the amount of protein that would be burned up from muscle each day, so that the muscle protein is maintained and the body is forced to go to fat as its principal fuel for energy. This approach has one additional benefit which is that adding protein to the diet in small amounts not only does not encourage weight gain, but also can be used by the body to manufacture glucose, the major fuel of the brain. By taking a small amount of protein during a reducing diet, you fuel your brain with glucose, which tends to counteract blood sugar problems which can result from diets, such as the high-fat diet, which do not supply a source of blood glucose. Glycogen, which is stored in the liver and muscles, is the major source of blood glucose. On any kind of a diet or fast, most of the glycogen is consumed within the first or second day. Without the extra protein, blood glucose would be difficult to manufacture at the levels required by the brain, and blood-sugar anomalies could result. You could develop symptoms of hypoglycemia (low blood sugar) with attendant central nervous system problems, such as mood swing, despondency, lethargy, depression, shakiness, and fatigue.

The theory behind the protein-sparing/partial-fasting diet is that when you follow this diet, your body is convinced that you are really serious about being on a fast, but you are tricking your body by supplying a small amount of protein. The basic way this diet is used is to eat no solid foods and to supply a small amount of dietary protein powder or liquid throughout the day. This diet received considerable attention a few years ago, but lost some of its supporters when it was found that some users of the diet died of heart-related medical problems. The protein supplements involved in these cases were deficient in certain essential nutrients, such as potassium and copper, essential amino acids such as tryptophan, and possibly magnesium and certain vitamins. More recently, protein powders which are derived from lacto-albumin or casein protein sources, rather than collagen, the major source of the earlier products, have become available. Collagen is a protein found in all connective tissue and is derived commercially from animal hides, which as you might imagine are not very biologically useful. You could eat a lot of gristle and shoe leather and still suffer from protein starvation. The newer protein powders and liquids derived from milk or egg protein are much more biologically utilizable, are well balanced, and may contain enrichment of vitamins and minerals necessary for its metabolism. This approach, then, which provides fifty grams of protein each day, will stimulate the body to use fat as its principal fuel for weight loss without wasting muscle. Lean body mass improves during the course of this type of diet when a healthful exercise routine is practiced.

A modification of this approach is to use a small amount of fructose each day as an appetite suppressant. Fructose, which is a sugar substance derived from corn syrup, will produce some appetite suppression, but it can easily be overused if taken too often during the day. Fructose in larger quantities can actually discourage weight loss, produce alterations of blood sugar, and raise various toxic elements within the blood. *No more than two or three teaspoons of fructose a day is acceptable.*

One important feature of the protein-sparing diet is that since the body thinks it is on a fast and stored fats are being mobilized for energy, the ketone level will increase in the blood. It has been found, however, that after three days, the brain actually clears its own ketones if you stay on this diet.

This would argue strongly that the protein-sparing diet is not appropriate for short-term use. The greatest benefit will occur if you stay on it three or more days. Staying on this diet for lesser periods of time will only encourage short-term muscle loss, and not the fat loss that is desired. If used, this dietary approach should be followed for a week at a time, thereby allowing the body an opportunity to adjust its metabolism and begin to use ketones as fuel. Even though there are some positive aspects of this diet, there are risks, and although it may be acceptable to follow a protein-sparing/partial-fast program for a week or so at a time *(never more than two weeks at a time)*, it should be done only when special circumstances exist. In my hospital programs, a "special circumstance" is determined by the client and the psychologist together, with the approval of the client's informed physician.

THE BOTTOM LINE

The bottom line questions on any diet are these:

1.   What is the quality of the weight you will lose during the course of the diet?
2.   How much stress will the diet put on your system as a result of ketone and acid buildup?
3.   Will the diet encourage higher levels of fitness and weight maintenance after it is broken?

Many of the diets that are currently promoted, although they will stimulate weight loss, will not encourage the right type of weight reduction, and may, in fact, be producing damaging effects to your health. You need to be aware that any kind of dietary regimen which employs fasting or modified fasting will be a biochemical shock to your body's machinery. This means that your system will be under more stress than when you are eating food. Therefore, to avoid trouble, you should be monitored closely by a physician or health practitioner who understands the dynamics of weight loss and physiology, as well as your psychological drives.

Remember, too, that once you have achieved your desired weight loss, you must be cautious in resuming normal eating patterns. Introducing heavy foods too quickly can be dangerous. Your body has made a transition to a new psysiology as a result of your dietary regime, and food should be reintroduced slowly so as not to overtax your metabolic machinery.

So, in summary, when you are in the bookstore looking for a "diet" book, remember: it's not the quantity of weight you lose that's so important, it's the quality of the weight that you lose and your attitudes about it. You want to find a weight-loss program that (1) does not put you in medical jeopardy; (2) that encourages weight loss mainly from fat stores, not from muscle mass or by dehydration through water loss; and (3) aids you in developing a greater belief in your own ability to determine your eating habits and your weight.

The purpose in discussing the five basic weight-loss diets into which all of the currently popular diets can be categorized is to point out that they hold no magic answers, and that their use requires a price in terms of health dangers, sometimes money and time, and *it is putting off learning what you need to know about your own capabilities to make more lasting changes and of dealing with the emotions that may be blocking these changes.*

Whether it's "Stillman's," "Atkins'," "Beverly Hills'," starch blockers, or the "Cambridge Diet," it makes no difference. You're playing around with your metabolic balance; trying to fool your body so you can eat large amounts of food, non-nutritional food, deleterious junk food, starve yourself in comfort, or avoid the effort of positive change, and **YOU'RE CHEATING YOURSELF.** You can go to the refrigerator because you need a hug, and a sweet snack distracts you from that need for a moment, but no weight-loss diet in the world is going to change that emotional need, unless it kills you. Many clients have acknowledged that they will keep right on eating when their stomach is so full it hurts. For the chronic food abuser, be it in the form of sporadic binges, constant snacking, voluminous portions at meals, hang-up food items, junk food, or, at the other end of the spectrum, eating next to nothing (anorexia), diets, in and of themselves, are not the answer to the problem. Inappropriate eating habits are most apt to be from a stimulus other than hunger. The likelihood of organic conditions within your body causing these urges are slim. The psycho/social are undoubtedly connected, but no weight-loss diet will change these.

A SIMPLE, HEALTHY, EFFECTIVE PLAN

When prospective clients learn that I have no magic diet to suggest, they are often disappointed. Some who are not ready to take advantage of a full program ask me if I won't give them a simplified program they can follow on their own. I give them the following weight-loss formula: (Note the similarities between the basic nutrition guidelines presented in Chapter 18, and the weight-loss program offered below)

1. Keep calorie consumption lower than expenditures.
2. Give up all red meat.
3. Add no salt to food, either during cooking or at the table.
4. Use whole-multi-grain sprouted bread made without flour or oil.
5. Give up all refined sugars. Use only small amounts of maple sugar, whole cane sugar, or honey if you must use a sweetener.

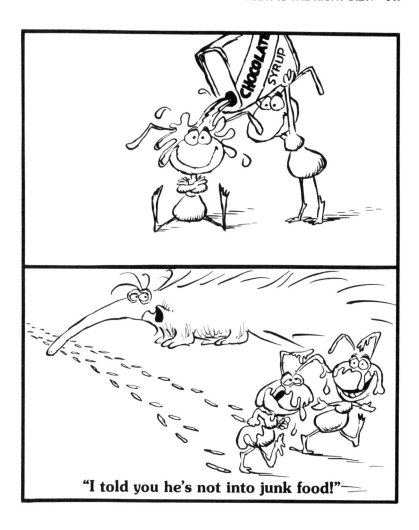

"I told you he's not into junk food!"

6. Drink 100% natural fruit juices (in small amounts) and vegetable juices, and 1/3 more pure fresh water than you are thirsty for. No alcohol.
7. Eat large amounts of fresh vegetables and sprouts and smaller amounts of fresh fruits.
8. Give up butter and margarines completely.
9. Eat beans and legumes that you prepare yourself.
10. Use yogurt, egg whites, low-fat, low-sodium cheeses and shelled nuts in small amounts.

11. Eliminate all packaged and processed foods from your diet.
12. Use balanced vitamin and mineral supplements.
13. In conjunction with the suggested diet, safely build your exercise routine to the point where you can comfortably do thirty to sixty minutes of aerobic exercise a day and have more usable energy as a result.

When I give the disappointed client this simple, spartan plan, he is, of course, even more dismayed. Certainly it must work, he agrees, but it sounds so harsh, impractical, and difficult. This plan offers no pretense of having your cake and eating it too. It is only simple, healthy, and effective. While it is true that some people have physical conditions which would make it unwise or difficult to jump into such a plan, I've seen individuals with many health problems thrive on variations of this program.

In most cases with which I'm familiar, the use of this type of health-oriented diet plan wasn't developed overnight. To suddenly make a radical change like this would lead to rapid burn-out in most overweight people. The people who are most comfortable with this dietary program have come to know their bodies intimately over a period of time. They are people motivated toward self-actualization, athletic excellence, health recovery, prevention of illness, discovering career potentials, etc. They are people looking for a higher quality of life, as well as life extension. Their diets vary from my simple plan — as they should — for each person's body is different. Lifestyles, ages, and goals are different. These people are from all walks of life, all income levels, all religious beliefs, and philosophies. They are all headed somewhere with their lives; they are not overweight, they don't smoke or drink, nor do they fear taking on or returning to these problems. Their focus and energy is on where they are headed, not where they have been.

What may be a surprise to you is that this wonderful group of people *"like"* what they eat. Their food preferences, like yours, have come from what they have been choosing. Their choices for healthful foods started because of what they wanted for their lives, and those choices soon became what they preferred. Their choices and preferences, like yours, will continue to change as their life needs and bodies change.

It is amazing how easily food preferences can change when you desire the change. Where the difficulty comes is in the resistance to change. If you sincerely desire a change, and the change can be achieved through different eating patterns, then you will be happy and comfortable eating the diet that will best effect the desired change. When a person on a weight-loss diet is in a constant struggle to follow a structured diet menu because they *HAVE* to, the chances for long-term change are poor. However, as soon as that same person quits struggling and opens up to change in learning to *like* new tastes, weight loss happens quickly. The opening up process happens more easily if you relax and have a forward-focused goal. As you begin making changes, based on information you have learned from classes, seminars, workshops, and books, practice listening to your body to hear its reactions to what you put into it. Developing this awareness takes time, practice, and, of course, interest. When your body reacts negatively, it tells you with sluggishness, discomfort, or any of a hundred-and-one other physical or psychological signs. The positive signs are just as important to pay attention to. Energy and alertness, a general feeling of well-being, creativeness, a sense of calm, clear eyes, sound teeth, lack of aches, pains, and rashes, etc. are clear indications that you're doing something right. Why wait for your physician to ask you about dramatic symptoms of serious health conditions that may have developed? Start listening to the messages you give yourself.

For the most part, you should build your own diet. You may, from time to time, need the guidance of a good nutritionist, but as a rule, you can come to be your own best nutritional advisor, with little need for weight-loss diets. We are only just beginning to learn of the potentials of healthful eating.

17

THE JOY OF
EXERCISE

Reducing your food intake below one thousand calories a day makes little sense unless you are hospitalized under a knowledgable doctor's care, and this would only be appropriate if your height/weight ratio had reached morbid proportions. For most people attempting weight loss, dropping nutritional intake significantly, without increasing exercise, will, at best, mean very slow *fat* loss. As I mentioned earlier, several pounds of water may come off very quickly, and lean muscle tissue will burn up two and one half times as fast as fat; however, this is *not* reduction of fat.

Without exercise to stimulate the Basic Metabolic Rate (BMR), when food intake is substantially reduced, the BMR slows down to protect the body as if it were starving, and it becomes very efficient at burning calories slowly. Prolonged exercise keeps the BMR up even while calorie intake is down, which assures the burning of fat while building lean muscle tissue for firming and shaping.

To be effective, exercise requires education, consistency, and commitment. It should be planned out according to what you wish to accomplish, and some very basic steps should be taken to assure success. It isn't only your body that is involved in exercise, but your mind and beliefs (spirit) as well.

SAFETY FIRST

When you select an exercise program, consider the following: you should be aware of your present physical limits, know how to do the exercise correctly, use quality equipment, and keep exercise in balance with the rest of your weight-loss program. If you are under thirty-five, no more than twenty percent above your ideal weight, have no current organic problems, and have no personal or family history of cardio-respiratory or alignment problems, you may want to use the guidelines set down for a safe start in Dr. Kenneth Cooper's book, *The Aerobic Way,* (Evans & Co., Inc., New York, New York). If you are over thirty-five, a medical stress test would be the best way to start, especially if you have a sedentary lifestyle.

The medical stress test is available in most communities. If there is more than one facility available, you may want to compare them for cost and factors included in the test. Both elements may vary a great deal from one provider to another. The equipment used by the provider and their experience using it could affect the quality and result of the test. Don't be afraid to ask questions and shop around. Providers that offer quality service want to tell you what's available.

Some of the tests that may be used during your stress exam to determine at what level of activity your exercise program should start are:

1. ***Treadmill E.K.G. (electrocardiogram)*** — measuring heart beat, pulse, and blood pressure.

2. ***Pulmonary check*** — measuring lung capacity for delivery of oxygen.

3. ***Body composition*** — measuring exact percentage of body fat by weighing you under water or through the use of recently developed electronic equipment. A calipers or pinch test may be used to determine percentage of body fat, but it is not as accurate.

4. ***Flexibility check*** — measuring potential injury areas for different activities.

5. **Strength/power** — measuring safe lifting or other activities requiring this capacity.
6. **Endurance** — measuring how long you can safely stay with an activity.
7. **Blood analysis** — measuring the red blood cells and amount of oxygen in the blood during exercise.

When you have an awareness of your maximum limits for safety and minimum limits for progress, you are closer to being ready to begin.

DO IT RIGHT

If exercise is done incorrectly, not only is much of its value lost, but also it could prove harmful or dangerous. Although exercise should be fun as well as a learning experience, it is also important to be serious about it and to develop the mental and emotional aspects of exercise as much as the physical movements. Books such as those by Jim Fixx, Mike Spino, and Dr. George Sheehan, can be very helpful. (see Bibliography.)

> **Once you are aware of your physical limitations, to be on the safe side, it is still important to know what exercise to select, where to do it, who to have instruct you, what the right equipment is, when and under what conditions to start and stop, as well as which activities will give you and your body the best chance for injury-free exercise over a prolonged period of time.**

Important factors, such as proper warm-up and cooldown, can make the difference between joy and love of exercise, and pain and medical bills. One of the reasons I did not fill this book with pictures of attractive people exercising, and descriptions of each exercise, is that I believe when you begin to exercise regularly, it is better to start off by being observed by a professional until you have mastered the performance of the exercise, with maximum safety for maximum benefit. Also, many of the exercises I could describe may not be the ones for you, suited to your interest, skill, or safety. After you know your limits, decide what you want to accomplish and which exercise options are open to you; then *you* select the activities and where and with whom to begin.

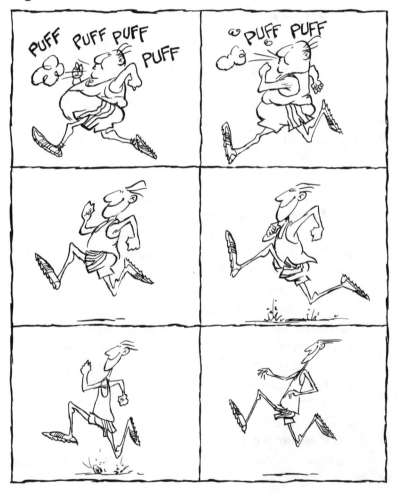

Some people overdo a good thing!

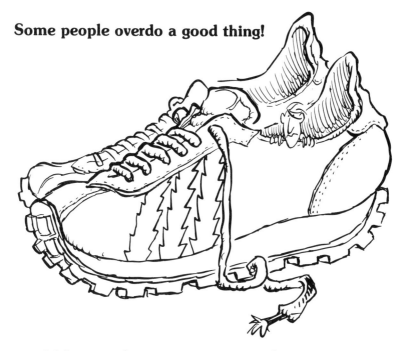

Make sure whatever program you select incorporates the following features:

1. **DAILY WORKOUT.** If you work a night shift, go on vacation, or the weather is bad, you should still do your exercise; it should become like brushing your teeth — part of your daily routine. After you have been exercising for six months or more, missing a day won't feel right. (Exercise that results from sports activity for entertainment, or physical activity which occurs as part of your job, is considered extra.) Ideally, your exercise should require little or no special equipment so that it can be done anywhere. You also need to be able to do it alone so that you don't have to depend on other people. It should be exercise that can be done indoors if the weather is bad. People that plan to swim or play tennis have too many reasons why they "can't do it today." Jogging, jumping rope, or bike riding afford less opportunity to cop out.

No matter which exercise you choose, you should warm up first, and that means *all* parts of your body. Your warm-up exercises can even serve as your "daily workout" if you do them vigorously enough. For me, warm-up exercise consists of a combination of yoga and calisthenics which I can do in an office, a motel room, or at home. This provides stretching and loosening of ligaments, joints, and muscle tissue, while massaging internal organs and firming stomach muscles, shoulders, arms, and legs. Doing these movements continuously, or with only a few seconds between sets, helps warm the body rapidly. I do these in the morning, virtually without fail. The complete set of exercises takes a half-hour. After the warm-up exercise, I either run or lift weights. If I have a lot of time, I may do both. Occasionally, I won't do either. It is very rare that I don't do at least the warm-ups, however. Weekends or vacations are fine times to play a sport, such as tennis, volleyball, ping-pong, or racket-ball or for skiing, hiking, or swimming. Sports like golf or bowling are fine for entertainment, but not for conditioning exercise. This may sound like a great deal of time to spend on exercising, but once you are in shape, you will see it as a nice balance with your other social, work, rest, and spiritual activities.

The *consistency* of your exercise is more important than your *proficiency*. When you work out daily over years of time, you realize how much a part of your lifestyle your exercise has become — something you take pride in and feel good about doing, rather than viewing it as a forced routine. When you feel that you are exercising only because you should, and you rigidly lock yourself into a routine, burnout or injury will be just around the corner. Burnout can happen to anyone; however, when exercise is being done out of satisfaction and desire, burnout, if it occurs at all, takes a much longer time to develop and is usually short lived.

To avoid burnout and to learn to *enjoy* your exercise, add variety — variety in your routine, kinds of exercise, where you exercise, with whom you exercise. Exercise with and without competition, vary the time of day; exercise alone or with a group. When I run, I even vary the kinds of strides and/or speed. Remember, exercise is psychological as well as physical, and burnout can be recognized as a depression or lack of energy. The mental part of exercise is very important, and we will discuss this more later.

Taking a day off now and then is fine, as long as you get right back to it. I don't recommend planning to take set days off, because it makes those days seem like rewards. Instead, be spontaneous with your off time; take days where emergency situations will not allow time to exercise, or you feel burnout may be setting in. Then get back to it as soon as possible. If you are making exercise the priority a healthy lifestyle requires, you will miss it very quickly and will want to get back to it soon.

2. **PROGRESSIVE EXERCISE.** Until you start approaching your peak condition, you should gradually increase the volume, intensity, speed, and level of difficulty of exercise. Deliberately try to extend yourself somewhat. Jogging a mile may be a challenge at first. Once you have jogged three miles several times, one mile holds little challenge.

Some people prefer to stagger their progression. For example, by jogging three miles one day, a mile-and-a-half the next time out, then three and a half miles the next time. Speed can be varied in the same manner. Once you approach your upper limits of exercise, you can start to adjust to a maintenance program. You may want to get into competition. Whether you choose to maintain or to compete, it is important to keep on learning and growing in your knowledge, skills, and use of exercise.

Most great athletes have come to realize that mental skills and self-awareness are as important to their achievement as physical skill and good training techniques. What you do with your mind concerning attitude, values, and concentration makes all the difference in the world when it comes to continuance and staying close to your peak. Learning how to meditate when you exercise has tremendous potentials and offers great advantage over straining to force your willpower to pull you through. Also, learn the best foods to eat in order to obtain the best results from exercise. Your assimilation and how you burn your food is an important factor. Again, it is important to recognize that you must deal with yourself as a whole person.

Being competitive in exercise takes a great deal more than simply maintaining for good health, and of course, the rewards and potential for injury are also greater. Competing with themselves to achieve their personal best time, greatest endurance, distance, or strength, is sufficient for many people and helps to keep interest levels high, while others crave competition with other people. For those of you who have this competitive drive, I truly recommend professional guidance or coaching. Read about the latest ideas on how to keep an edge and prime yourself physically and mentally, as well as how to prepare yourself for those times when you will fall short of your goal. Injury or depression can kill your interest in an exercise very rapidly. With good preparation, mental and physical, your progress can go on indefinitely.

3. **BALANCED EXERCISE.** As I advocate in all other aspects of your life, balance in your exercise is important. Balance means breaking down exercise into three main categories: stretching, cardiorespiratory, and contractual exercise.

* *Stretching* is loosening and pulling joints, ligaments, and muscles gently, slowly, and firmly. Yoga and ballet movements are good examples of disciplines that heavily emphasize stretching.
* *Cardiorespiratory (aerobic) exercise* increases your heart rate, pulse rate, basic metabolic rate, breathing,

and blood pressure. Once the healthy heart rate is elevated, it should remain so for a prolonged period of time (30-60 minutes, 3-6 times a week). This will build your lung power, strengthen your heart muscle, improve your circulation, nourish your cells, increase your endurance, burn calories, and improve your energy level.

* *Contractual exercise* firms the body by working muscles against muscles or against dead weight or fixed objects. This is used to shape the body and define and build muscle mass. Pushups, pullups, and squats are good examples of calisthenic-type exercise that will help in firming your muscles. Body-building machines and weights can be purchased or used in exercise facilities. Building (changing inches) and firming your muscles improves your self-image and confidence as you gain greater control of your body and feel new strength and endurance levels.

Within these three categories of exercise fall many different types of activities, including the following:

Badminton	Hockey	Skating
Baseball	Jumping rope	Skiing
Basketball	Martial arts	Soccer
Biking	(Judo, Karate,	Softball
Body building	Akido, Ta'i	Swimming
Calisthenics	Chi, etc.)	Tennis
Dance	Mountain climbing	Track and
Fencing	Paddle boating	field events
Football	(rowing)	Volleyball
Handball	Racketball	Walking
Hiking	Running	Wrestling

Some of these are team sports, and some are individual, but they are all forms of exercise that can improve the way you experience the world physically and mentally.

CHOOSING AN INSTRUCTOR

After you have taken a stress test to determine your present physical condition, you may wish to have some guidance in the exercise activities you have selected. Often this is only needed in the beginning stages or periodically during your program. If you do not already have a fundamental knowledge of the activity, it is wise to read up on the subject prior to contacting an instructor. This will save time with the instructor; you will learn faster and more easily; and your questions will be fewer and more pertinent to your individual needs.

Where, when, and from whom you receive guidance can vary a great deal. The main sources providing qualified instructors are:

1. YMCA and YWCA
2. City Parks and Recreation Programs
3. Adult evening courses at public high schools and colleges.
4. Hospitals with health activities and sports medicine departments.

These facilities and programs usually are low-cost, offering a large variety of activities, set class times, and graded levels of skills for various groups.

Other places offering lower-cost classes, but with less assurance of quality guidance and, most often, a more limited selection of activities, are:

1. Free universities (non-credit courses run by students at a state university)
2. Church programs
3. Private clubs
4. Large business employee programs

Sometimes these programs are more convenient, require less trouble, offer the opportunity to exercise with friends, and may even be free. The following places to exercise could have top quality instructors or some with no training credentials at all. Instructors in these facilities often serve more as sales personnel or motivators than educators. With the following types of exercise facilities, it is always wise to check credentials, equipment, and program offerings, as well as financial rating with the Better Business Bureau.

1. Private or membership spas
2. Commercial spas (chains)
3. Apartment complex recreation facilities/spas
4. Fraternal/social clubs
5. "Fat farms" (exclusive)

In some of the above facilities, no instruction at all is offered. The equipment may be in poor repair and inadequate for heavy group use. Overall quality could swing from one extreme to another, depending upon the efforts of the current management. Talking with several people who use the facility will usually give you the answers you need.

Yet another place to consider might be a hospital or rehabilitation clinical therapy facility designed for people whose special physical problems require special instruction and equipment. Also, if it is appropriate and affordable, tutoring from an exercise physiologist or from sports training health resorts catering to top-line athletes and celebrities are options. For the average person, these places are not necessary. Again, whenever you employ any specialist's advice, check out his credentials, academic training, background, experience, and references (including recent client reference).

If you are seeking training from an instructor in a specialized exercise activity such as martial arts, remember that just because an instructor is highly skilled in one physical discipline does not necessarily qualify him to give training in other sports or exercise activity. It can be a mistake to take advice from a person on subjects outside his field of expertise.

EXERCISE EQUIPMENT

Some equipment can be helpful to your exercise program. Purchasing quality equipment for a spare room is fine, *if* you use it. Generally speaking, we get what we pay for, and it might seem that you should buy the most elaborate and expensive equipment available if you are really serious about an exercise program. However, the fine, chrome-plated equipment sold for commercial use is not necessary for personal home use. Although some excellent universal gym equipment is on the market, it requires space and expense which most of us cannot afford. It is not necessary to have a special piece of equipment for each individual exercise. A few quality pieces designed for home use are adequate to supplement complete daily workouts. Extra equipment has no real value except the temporary psychological motivation stemming from the sales pitch.

The main things you should have at home are (1) a good thick rug or padded mat so you won't bruise yourself when you do floor exercises; (2) some type of weight lifting equipment; and (3) a jump rope or possibly a stationary bicycle or rowing machine. Much of the rest is more than necessary.

If your budget will allow, you might want to purchase one of the reasonably priced quality home gym sets on the market. Some are very complete and can be time saving. One of the best low-cost, versatile, safe, and effective portable gym units is the *Lifeline Gym*, manufactured in Madison, Wisconsin by Lifeline Products & Marketing, Inc. This gym equipment has a great aerobic feature for building endurance. It is also excellent for athletes' special needs or for physical rehabilitation. Again, however, with a good balanced program, this equipment is not mandatory.

CLOTHING AND SHOES

As for special clothing, little should be necessary for most useful sports (sports that are not just for socializing). Two main things to keep in mind when purchasing clothing for sport are: it should allow for freedom of movement without being so loose as to be hazardous, and it should protect your body without contributing to excess heating or chilling. *Gortex* and other similar materials on the market are especially good for runners' clothes.

When footwear is being considered, the best advice I can give is to get the best you can afford for a particular type of activity. It isn't necessary to purchase expensive racing shoes if you are only doing general conditioning; but *if you are running regularly, the quality of your footwear is very important.* It is possible to get good, specific footwear advice in many of the sports magazines, from school athletic instructors, podiatrists, athletic medicine professionals, or even from some specialty stores that handle a good line of athletic shoes.

THE MENTAL / PSYCHOLOGICAL ASPECT OF EXERCISE

As I mentioned previously, the mental or psychological aspect of exercise is extremely important for multiple reasons. In dealing with weight problems, it is commonly necessary to change attitudes about exercise in order for it to become an activity that is looked forward to rather than dreaded. The chapters on changing, procrastination, and motivation are very important in this respect. For the overweight person who has a history of a sedentary lifestyle, the idea of changing attitudes about exercise is initially more important than the exercise itself.

Getting into exercise means letting go of the struggle between thinking one *should* and emotionally *talking oneself out of it.* It may mean using imagery and desensitization, meditation and/or self-hypnosis. For the most part, it need only mean opening up to exercise — a simple decision not to push yourself to like or dislike it, only to experience it in the prescribed way. If, in addition to this, you have made the decision to include exercise in your life — for the rest of your life — then it becomes a matter of finding how it can best fit in. Your body was made to move; it functions best when you exercise regularly. So, if you will simply let down your defenses against exercise and stop predetermining why you won't like it, you will go a long way toward learning how to like it. Certainly, if you've decided to exercise at 5:30 A.M., and you got to bed at 12:30 A.M., you will quickly teach yourself to dislike exercise. Most things will not seem good when you are too exhausted to enjoy them. By employing some logical steps, with your defenses down, you can come to love exercise, and in return, your body will love you for it.

World-class athletes who become champions are able, in one way or another, to have an *intense focus* (without straining) on the physical feat they are performing; yet, they are making a *relaxed effort.* Mental imagery is brought into play, and these athletes may feel as though they are in harmony with everything around them. They may feel at times, as though they are in a slow motion movie, and are able to anticipate exactly where all the action is going on; they may even feel they have control over a ball in flight. These peak experiences occur when concentration, belief, and physical skills all come together in a single event. Muscles are in total synchronization with the environment, as the mind is with the body. Peak experiences are fully in the "now;"

yesterday's mistakes and tomorrow's fantasies are not present. This kind of total absorption is more than mental distraction. It is an experience of harmony with the world and everything in it. To condition the mind at the same time as the body brings out the ultimate athlete in each of us. We learn to let go of our resistance and flow with our world.

Learning to practice meditation in many ways and in many settings can contribute greatly to realizing peak experiences. The "runner's high," which I've experienced on many occasions, usually comes after I've been focusing inward on my own body movement. I go from simple sensations to euphoric feelings of lightness, smoothness, and the suspension of time — a sense of freedom, balance, and energy that makes all the usual movement almost effortless; and the best part of it is that you don't have to win a gold medal to experience this.

SUMMARY

With exercise, as in other areas of your life, decisions about changes in your lifestyle are left to you. You now have a basic guide and you know where to seek additional advice and instruction. The details are up to you. If you do not decide to make exercise a *permanent part* of your lifestyle, it may be better not to start at all. Just like going up and down on the weight scale, it may do more harm than good. But if you do decide to pursue an exercise program as a permanent part of your lifestyle, the advantages are unlimited. Your attitude will change from viewing exercise as a boring, painful chore to seeing it as an exciting, fulfilling, energy power source of pride and accomplishment.

The sooner you become consistent, without being rigid, in your exercise program, the faster you will develop, and the sooner you'll realize the benefits. Rigidity in your pattern of exercise will cause stress, just as it would in all other aspects of your holistic program. Learning to flex and roll with your program while being consistent and meeting the other needs of your daily life is the goal to strive for. If you are going to compete in the exercise of your choice, my suggestion is to compete with yourself and to keep the competition realistic, or the joy of it all may be lost.

Meditation can also play a part in your exercise program. As you begin to reach your upper limits, stress levels will be reduced, and the overall experiences will be enhanced by employing meditative techniques. If exercise is going to pay off for you, it is necessary to do more than simply go through the motions.

It is up to you now. All the magic motivation you require is there inside you. *Remember, energy begets energy.* Once you're in shape you will add hours of energy to your day.

18

PUTTING IT ALL TOGETHER

The fact that you are willing to set up your own program is very significant. It is a statement about you. It says that you are making an organized effort and that you are willing to take responsibility for yourself. I may be your guide, but you are doing the work — making decisions and accepting the responsibility for putting them into action. If these steps are true for you, it says that you are willing and able to change an old attitude. You no longer have to say, "That's just the way I am."

SETTING UP YOUR PROGRAM

> **The program you are getting ready to set up is one based on a holistic health/wellness model which can be summed up as body-mind-spirit, or physical fitness (exercise), proper nutrition, psychological/mental health, environment and stress management — with self responsibility for all of it.**

As you approach setting up your own program, it will be necessary for you to use the guidance material presented in this book and apply it to your own life situation. You will need to rearrange your priorities, possibly dropping some activities as you add others. It will take time, effort, energy, and may cost some money. If you manage your program effectively, you will go slowly at the beginning so you will not feel overwhelmed. This will be added assurance of success. As you progress, your speed of change and momentum can increase. Each part of your program will affect all of the other parts. No part has to come either first or last, and it is possible to work on all parts at the same time as long as you are realistic about how much you attempt. Working with other people — professionals, peers, friends, and relatives, is fine as long as *you* continue to be the decision maker and to accept responsibility for what you do and how you do it. If you go slowly and consistently, you will succeed at most of what you attempt; however, this will involve some trial and error. When things get difficult for you, it is important that you don't put yourself down. You must give yourself permission not to be perfect — to say, "that's OK" and start over with a new effort. At times you may feel bored or depressed, and that is where a support group comes in. Maybe you even need to let some efforts go for awhile and then come back to those things later.

> **If you *open up* to your program rather than *force* yourself through it, your effort will be much smoother and more successful.**

When you incorporate other programs into your plan, such as a weight-loss club, be careful not to let their goals dominate your own. Take what you want—whatever fits into your program — and leave the rest. How organized and structured your program becomes is up to you. The only question is how can you be most effective in working toward your goal? Many people find it helpful to keep a daily journal or log in order to chart their progress. Actually seeing your success stimulates greater effort.

Making the decisions involved in formulating a detailed plan is almost as important as the plan itself, for several reasons:

1. Because you are a unique individual and should know your own special needs better than anyone else.
2. Because the more you run your own program, the better you feel about yourself.
3. Your effort will add to your self-awareness (identity), just as driving your own car helps you to know your way around better than if someone is chauffering you.
4. Learning self-responsibility is what wellness is all about.
5. Creativity, imagination, and innovation, which are useful to all of the life-adjustment process, can be developed.

Making your program a priority in your time schedule (should I go to my friend's party or to my encounter group?) is absolutely necessary to success. The lower the priority your wellness program receives on a day-to-day basis, the slower your progress will be, and the less you will trust yourself. What you *do* in this regard is much more important than what you *write down* on the paper you are using to organize and plan your effort. As soon as you make sound priority judgements spontaneously, you will realize that your program doesn't have to be as organized.

Remember, it is also important not to be rigid in your program or to expect perfection. This will put a strain on you and you are likely to burn out quickly. What you are aiming for is a relaxed, balanced effort so that you can make adjustments easily as you go.

One of the best ways I know to assure success in your effort is to become a leader of others along the very same lines. Your family, or even one friend, can serve in this regard. You will never learn more or be more consistent than when you teach, or better yet model, what you wish to teach. Let's get started now with assessment and attitude.

ASSESSING YOUR CURRENT STATUS

Assess Your Attitude

Assessing your attitude is the first step in setting up your holistic program. Because attitudes are very much related to your beliefs and values, the success of your whole program may be determined by your willingness to view your attitudes objectively and change those which need changing. The changes will not all take place the second you recognize the need to change, but if the awareness and commitment are there, as you go through your program changing your behavior, your attitudes will gradually change also.

Answer *Yes* or *No* to the following questions:

1. Do you know you can change? _____
2. Are you able to be honest with yourself? _____
3. Are you able to be open about yourself with special others? _____
4. Can you let down your defenses enough to be reasonably *objective* about yourself? _____
5. Do you actively seek out positive change in yourself? _____
6. Do you believe you are responsible for your own change? _____
7. Do you believe you are at least half responsible for what you are now as a person? _____

8. Do you know you can commit yourself to an effort and stay with it to completion or until you are sure that the effort is either unproductive or counter-productive? ____
9. Is your attitude determined by you, rather than by other people or circumstances? ____
10. Do you believe your freedom to change is continuous throughout your life? ____

If you can easily answer "yes" to all of the above questions, you are probably in a good mental state to continue with setting up your program. If any of your answers are "no" or "maybe," further change is needed before you begin. Get feedback about your attitudes from special people in your life as well as from your support group. If you don't have a support group, find out about how to get into one later in this chapter. It is also possible to take a personal written inventory at a counseling or testing center, with focuses on attitude. One of the better inventories is the *Personal Orientation Inventory* (POI), by Everett Shostrum.

Once you know you have a good handle on what your attitudes are and what needs to be changed, set up a plan to make those changes and proceed. From time to time during your program, especially when the going is slow or difficult, return to the ten questions you just answered and review them.

Assess Your Physical Condition

Assessing your physical condition is also an extremely important task before starting a holistic weight program. Being aware of just exactly what your individual strengths and weaknesses are will help a great deal in knowing what can be expected in all other areas of your program. As mentioned in the previous chapter, many universities and some private clinics have set up stress testing equipment to give measurements of all vital signs during activity, instead of before and/or after exercise. Computers give feedback that is very clear in establishing safe guidelines for you. This, coupled with a general physical examination utilizing lab measurements, will give you a lot of information and reassurance. In addition to these tests, I highly recommend completing an inventory of your level of wellness. *The WISE Indicator©* (Wellness Inventory and Stress Education), which I developed together with Scott Rigden, M.D., is such a program, whereby you can assess your level of wellness. The inventory is used to examine your lifestyle as it relates to your health. In the future this type of assessment may prove to be more valuable than the annual physical in determining and preventing illness, as well as a kick-off point toward good health. For more information about *The WISE Indicator©*, write to the Human Dynamics Institute, 3605 N. 7th Ave., Phoenix, AZ 85013, or contact Health Plus Publishers.

Again, as mentioned earlier, if you are no more than twenty percent above your ideal weight, have no personal or family history of organic problems, no existing symptoms, and feel that you cannot afford a stress test and physical exam, you may want to use the "step test" in Dr. Cooper's book, *The Aerobic Way,* in conjunction with *The WISE Indicator©.* Naturally, if you should discover any cautionary information in any of these measurements, seek professional consultation as to the best and safest way to proceed. *Possible problem areas should not be used as reasons (excuses) to give up on your program.* They should simply alert you to potential problems and the fact that you may need to make some adjustments or modifications in your plan.

Assess Your Living and Working Situations

To assess your current living and working situations, a time outline of your activities is a good place to begin. In this part of your assessment, you are attempting to find spare time in which to fit parts of your program. For example, time spent in unproductive or counterproductive activity can be restructured. This is not to say that you should become a compulsive, rigid clock watcher or never have any fun; rather it is a matter of becoming more aware and getting into more positive self-development. This will result in increased flexibility, spontaneity, creativity, and a sense of adventure. As the people close to you watch you change, they may feel confused, frightened, angry, or amused at first. Hopefully the end result of your change is that you will become more exciting, interesting, and respected by them. Be prepared for the likelihood that your circle of friends may change. Some of your old friends may fade away as new ones who are attuned to your new lifestyle and attitudes enter your life. At times you may feel guilty that you're letting people down because you don't live up to their old expectations the way you used to. Don't feel guilty. This is the way it should be.

> **You're becoming a new person — one *you* like, and everybody whose life you touch will benefit from it.**

The reason to feel guilty is gone! The point is, as soon as you outline your use of time and interactions, begin to take a relaxed, open look at where and how you can fit in parts of your program all day and even all night — yes, even your dreams and the proper kind of rest can work for you.

Work is often seen as so important to survival that it can easily be given priority over everything else in our lives. Many divorced people and early-life heart attack victims can attest to this. Some organization and business leaders are starting not only to become aware of the futility of single dimension lives, but also to see the dollar value in countering workaholic attitudes. Visionary leaders are setting up assistance programs to aid their employees in seeking and finding healthier holistic lifestyles. Workshops, seminars, smoking and weight programs, counseling groups, and exercise programs are being offered by employers. You may want to take steps to initiate a program of this kind where you work. Many professionals such as myself are available to help organizations that wish to develop employee assistance programs, and the profit returns have proven to be substantial and varied. Those employee assistance programs which pay off the best, in terms of lower absenteeism, less injuries, increased productivity, etc., include exercise facilities, counseling on healthful nutrition, and the time and opportunity as well as incentive to utilize the benefit. In addition, many companies offer a health insurance benefit package that rewards employees for staying well.

Some changes you can make will be obvious, such as where and how to spend your lunch hour. It may be that you can fit in some brief exercise, a meditation period, eating at a natural food restaurant, or, at the very least, engaging in supportive or confrontational conversations with another person who is also seeking personal growth and development. Certainly, reading material related to self-growth is always a possibility. You need to look at every aspect of your life, with whom you are spending it, and what the outcome is. Some facets of your life you may like, and even savor, even though you know they work against you. You may feel you'd be overwhelmed if you made too many changes at once. You may think you are making a few tough changes so you deserve to keep a few old vices. You may feel defensive, or that there are certain things about you that you just are not ready to change at this time. If this is what is going on in your head as you assess your situation, then we are right back to attitude. Certainly everyone has some things about themselves that they may never benefit by changing; however, in this assessment state, all parts of you and the way you spend your time should be examined as *possibilities* for change. It is true that you can't change everything at once, and you don't want to overwhelm yourself. However, it is also true that you need to continually challenge and push yourself a little. *Openness, honesty, objectivity, and feedback are absolutely mandatory to change.* Hanging on to the old you will only interfere with change. If you want to go somewhere new and be someone new in the future, then let go of an equal amount of the past. None of your changes need to be thought of as permanent. You can always go back to being fat. Finding something new, exciting, and lovable in yourself will more than take the place of anything that you give up. Some things will become easier and more fun. Right now, just starting to examine what you are doing with every minute — with your kids, parents, friends, spouse, on the job, at church, at school — is important. Your potential resources are many: people, time, skills, talents, intelligence, education, science, beliefs, groups, energy, health, work, needs, challenges, and problems. All depend on how you look at them.

> **Even problems can become opportunities to like yourself. If everything were perfect for you, and you had no cares, concerns, or challenges, how could you ever demonstrate to yourself that you have worth?**

Isn't meeting a challenge or overcoming a fear the way to find happiness? Each time you confront a fear or resolve a problem, it opens doors for new possibilities. In this way life is always new, always an adventure, instead of stagnant, life-less, depressing and boring. Remind yourself, "If I'm bored, it is because I'm a bore." Boredom is a state of anxiety — fear of opening up or letting go.

Assess Your Nutritional Status

Becoming aware of your nutritional intake, assessing your metabolism and vitamin, mineral, and protein needs is an extremely important matter which requires your continu-ing attention for the rest of your life. This may sound difficult at first, but once it becomes a part of your lifestyle (just like overeating was) it is easy — and it doesn't take that much time. A lot of what you are going to need to know will come from sensing your body's reactions to what you put into it. By listening to your body carefully, you will gradually begin to pick up on what it has been telling you all along. You not only start to sense what is happening internally, but also you start to observe and get feedback on symptoms of behavior and moods coming to the outside. Reading texts and attend-ing classes, workshops, and seminars on nutrition will help you to become a better listener and observer of yourself.

Few M.D.'s have training in nutrition; health food store clerks are seldom qualified to make recommendations; dieticians may come out of home economics schools which teach a traditional and sometimes narrow-viewed approach to nutrition; and within the natural food school of thought, a lot of controversy exists between different authorities. Find-ing the right professional is difficult, but for special needs and concerns, such as existing health problems and symptoms, you may feel a need to do so at some point. To provide the best assurance that you will receive adequate and correct counseling, you should choose a professional nutritionist who fits the following profile:

* A person with at least a master's degree in nutrition, and preferably a Ph.D. in nutrition-focused biochemistry.
* A person who is not radical in his or her concepts of nutrition.
* A person who takes a balanced, holistic approach to nutrition, health, and life.
* A person who is an example of what he or she professes.
* Ideally, a person who has training in a related field, such as medicine or psychology.
* A person who has a good track record among others he or she has served.
* A person who will devote the time and attention necessary to understand you.

If you wish to have a specific nutritional assessment of your body, testing can be done in the laboratory with blood, feces, urine, skin and hair analysis to determine what is coming *out* of you after the technicians have assessed what went *in*. This, of course, is not always constant — your body changes with time, stress and lifestyle — but it gives you a good starting place. To have this testing done, seek out professionals and get their interpretations of the results. In the meantime, use the following nutrition guidelines if your health is relatively good and stable:

1. Eat a balanced diet which includes a wide variety of healthful foods.
2. Substitute fresh foods for canned and packaged foods whenever possible. Frozen foods are preferable to canned if fresh foods are not available.
3. When possible, eat organically grown foods (foods grown without the use of harmful chemical fertilizers or insecticides).

4. Increase the amount of vegetables, fruits, legumes, and seeds, with careful use of dairy products (preferably skim milk) and nuts in small amounts.
5. Keep oils and fats to a minimum.
6. Keep red meat to a minimum.
7. Eliminate all refined sugars from your diet.
8. Add no salt to your food.
9. Stay away from food additives. Eat simple, clean food.
10. Avoid caffeine, alcohol, and tobacco.
11. Log your food intake for at least one week every third month.
12. Breakfast should be your main meal. Eat lighter meals the rest of the day, particularly at dinnertime.
13. If you want to lose weight, eat fewer calories than you burn.

With practice listening to your body and study of the subject of nutrition, you will learn what is healthy and natural for your body. If you follow a holistic program, you will lose weight and learn to make necessary adjustments as you go. Somebody else's magic diet will not come to save you. Focus your energy on total, healthy development.

Now is a good time to clean out the junk and restock your cupboards. If it is possible to gain full cooperation from your family on the idea of having only nutritional food in your home, it will be a good deal easier to start eating a natural, healthful array of foods. If it is not possible to gain their cooperation, then set up a special cupboard and a special section of the refrigerator just for your use.

The idea is simple, if junk food (and excessive amounts of any food) are not readily available, you will be less likely to eat them. Rid yourself of all refined sugar and overprocessed foods, white breads, and packaged foods. Stock up on natural, clean foods (unprocessed or minimally-processed foods that are as fresh as possible and have been properly stored and handled). You'll find a good cool pantry and refrigerator are needed to store foods that aren't full of preservatives. Clean food does not have preservatives, imitation colorings, fillers, stabilizers, taste enhancers, or any additives — only the natural food, the way it was meant to be eaten. Some packaged foods are more chemical than food. Become a label reader and know what you are eating. Once you learn to understand what your body needs, see to it that you get it in the best forms, in amounts you can handle.

The foods you want in your kitchen are:

* fresh vegetables
* fruits
* whole-grain breads (flourless, if possible)
* a few dairy products (skin milk, low-fat cottage cheese, natural white brick cheeses, no-fat yogurt) — dairy products are optional
* eggs — optional
* mixed, uncracked or freshly shelled nuts, in small amounts
* seeds, in small amounts
* legumes
* beans
* herbs and spices
* honey, raw sugar, or maple sugar (use in small amounts)
* fruit juices, in limited amounts
* pastas, rice, potatoes, and other starches

If you eat meat, do so in small amounts and stay as much with sea food and skinless clean fowl as possible. If you feel you must eat red meat, make sure it is as lean as possible (veal), and if you can get fresh meat that is not full of nitrates, hormones, and colorings, you'll do much better. Once you learn what good food is and have your cupboard and refrigerator full of it, you can concentrate on appetizing menus and recipes. The bookstores abound with cookbooks, as do popular women's and fitness magazines.

Supplements such as vitamins and minerals are good insurance that you are getting the nutrients you need. How much you take will depend on your activity, level of stress, and food intake, as well as other factors. *Vitamins & Minerals: The Health Connection,* by Anni Airola Lines, R.D. (Health Plus Publishers, Phoenix, AZ, 1985) is a good guide to follow regarding vitamin and mineral use. If you do use vitamin and mineral supplements, take them together, with meals. The individualized details of supplementation should be developed through personal study and learning to sense your own body's needs, along with the help of professionals such as nutritionists or holistically-oriented physicians. (For a more detailed discussion of the "right diet," see Chapter 16.)

Career Evaluation

Your work is a major part of your life. No single activity requires more of your time except sleep. Major portions of your self-worth, self-esteem, and respect from others come from your work. Your income level, prestige, friends, mate, education, home, leisure, etc., all are usually closely related to your occupation. Because of this, your emotions, and thus your happiness, are heavily influenced, both personally and as family units, by what you do for a living. With these facts in mind, you cannot overlook your career when setting up a program to eliminate obesity from your life.

To assess your work situation effectively may take more time and energy and cause more inconvenience than you wish to deal with; however, even if you end up deciding that you are in the best career situation right now, you will be pleased that you went through the process, and you'll be more attuned to and ready for needed changes when the time comes. Consider taking the following steps in assessing your career:

1. Read two or three current books on careers and life planning.
2. In career centers at colleges, Veterans' Administration centers, and employment services, take a battery of inventory tests dealing with personality, job interest, values and attitudes, academic and special skill tests.
3. Have professionals administer, score, and interpret the inventories for you.
4. Review general career reference books, such as the *Dictionary of Occupational Titles,* found in libraries and government employment offices.
5. With feedback from significant persons in your life, assess your future needs and wants for income, living circumstances, marriage, children, lifestyle, avocations, and beliefs. Allow for your own growth.
6. Assess the price of change — stress in transition, geographical moves, further education, temporary or permanent decrease in income, loss of status, the continued needs of other persons in your life.
7. Measure the position you now have, with its merits and problems, against the possibilities of change to other careers or other positions within your current career area.

If you determine that a career change would be of potential benefit, many more steps should be taken in assessing the job requirements and opportunities, your skills, need for additional training, and the means of entering into the new line of work. Assistance from a career specialist could be most valuable to you in this change process. One suggestion is to start at a state college, employment office, or the VA as soon as you complete your reading on the subject. These services should be of little or no cost.

IMPORTANT ASPECTS
OF YOUR PROGRAM

Relaxation

Relaxation techniques can be extremely important to you and your program, and should be allowed for on a daily basis. Many, many techniques are available to you, and the one that works best for you will be the one you believe in. In this chapter, I will only touch on the subject of relaxation. For detailed information, see Chapter 9, "The Stress Factor."

Meditation and self-hypnosis are probably the most popular relaxation techniques and hold the most potential. Other techniques, such as biofeedback, require equipment and money, but if it works for you, it will be worth it. The principles of relaxing are much the same in all techniques, and once they are clear to you, you may want to devise or formulate your own personal, innovative technique. Knowing you've been creative often adds to your success.

Some relaxation techniques, such as self-hypnosis, Ta'i Chi, and yoga, will be more effective with professional guidance, therefore, I have selected a meditation technique here which you can easily do on your own. Again, hundreds of meditation techniques are available, and the one method I've selected is no more the "best" than any other. Only the method that you accept and use effectively and regularly is the best one for you.

One Method of Meditation

1. Set your alarm clock or kitchen timer for thirty minutes.
2. Seat yourself in a firm, straight-backed chair with hands on your lap, palms up, legs uncrossed, and feet flat on the floor.

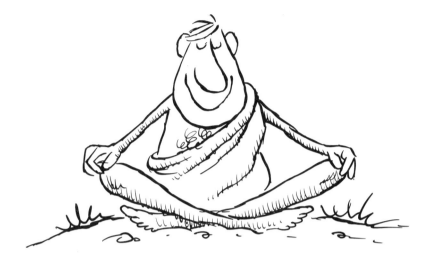

Meditating On You

3. Permit your eyes to close and begin to focus on your out breath (just your breath going out).
4. Count each breath for its full length. "O...n...e..."
5. Count only up to three, then return to one.
6. Accept your breath in any manner it comes out, short or long.
7. Visualize the number you're counting in your mind's eye.
8. Choose a time for meditation when your stomach is not too full, and when you are wide awake. Attempting to meditate on a full stomach will work against you. If you are very fatigued when you meditate, you'll probably only go to sleep.
9. Accept that if your mind should wander while you meditate, you simply return to your focus of counting.

10. Practice daily, and you will soon realize greater self-awareness, calmness, energy, peace of mind, and a growing ability for emotional and physical control. Consistent practice is more important than how perfect your meditation is.

Exercise

Setting up an exercise program was deserving of a full chapter (Chapter 17, "The Joy of Exercise"), and worth additional mention here. No self-development effort, and certainly no weight-loss program of any merit at all, will be without an exercise regime. The physical, emotional, and spiritual benefits of exercise are tremendous. It goes far beyond building muscles and looking good — not that I wish to play these benefits down. The health and fitness of your body is frequently in proportion to the health and fitness of your mind. Your concern for your body will hopefully go beyond physical fitness to high-level wellness (that state where your natural immunity system functions near its peak). Your body is up front representing you, the person, at all times. It has as much influence on your energy levels, moods, attitudes, alertness, calmness, etc., as your mind does. Your body is involved in every aspect of your life, including the most intellectual activities, all of the time.

Exercise helps your body function at its peak for long periods of time without breakdowns. Exercise is needed not only for your weight-loss program, but also to maintain good health, and the sooner you accept and include exercise in your lifestyle, the sooner it will stop being boring and painful. Once you accept and practice exercise daily, progressively, and in a balanced manner for six months to a year, it will become as necessary and important to you as brushing your teeth. It can become fun, exciting, and a source of pride, rewards, compliments, and challenge. It is much more natural than sitting and watching the 'boob tube" or hanging over the bar in a smoke-filled room. Exercise can provide "highs," get you in touch with new feelings, and it can lead to a greater sense of control over your own destiny. It certainly is a learning process and, I feel, a measurement of strength, intelligence, and stability.

Sexual Development

To have a full balance in your program, you should include your sexual development. Sex could have been included with exercise, but it's more than just exercise, of course. It could have been a part of interpersonal relations and love, or communicating, or assessing your circumstances or resources. Because it could have been a part of so many other things, I believe it deserves a place of its own.

Sex is biological, psychological, sociological, and spiritual. It is sensual in a way equal to eating — if not more so. It burns up calories via aerobic exercise; it is as calming as any tranquilizer. It can give you a sense of fulfillment, sharing, of being loved and loving, as well as a biological release. It is a tremendous gift. (And we are not usually ingesting calories when we enjoy it!)

Sex deserves a place of balance in your life, and you can develop sexually, as well as in other ways. Your sexual potential is unlimited as to quality and variety, and you need not lose it as you age.

Sexual development includes: attitudes, total sensitivity, imagination, creativity, intuitiveness, and appreciation. Like an athlete learning to make a relaxed effort to achieve new peaks or find new meaning in old ones, learn to get away from intellectualizing so that you can live, in the moment, with full sensual abandon. Learn to accept and exercise your fantasies, appreciate and develop your body, its suppleness, and energy.

The following tips can assist you in developing your sexual potentials:

1. Read the *Joy of Sex,* or a book by Masters and Johnson.
2. Develop your physical fitness level.
3. Learn how to relax or "let go." (Use relaxation techniques such as meditation)
4. Practice fantasizing erotic scenes that stimulate you.
5. With the help of a counselor or a close friend, work through old inhibiting messages or guilt feelings from your youth and previous relationships.
6. Stimulate all of your senses with smells, tastes, sounds, colors, and textures — practice titillating your senses to bring them to peak sensitivity.
7. Add variety to sexual encounters with new settings, positions, time of day, etc., or, if appropriate, a new partner.
8. With a special, cared for, or loved partner, create an atmosphere such as the following for communication exercise: After a stimulating light meal by candlelight, turn on some easy background music and disrobe each other. While you are completely nude, use some scented body lotion or oil, and take turns giving each other a slow, easy body massage. The person giving the massage does not talk, and the person receiving the massage talks only of his or her hopes, dreams, and goals for the future. When both partners have had a full massage, continue the tactile experience in a warm bubble bath and whatever may follow. Experiences and efforts such as these, even as infrequently as once a month, can make the difference between pleasant, brief encounters and reaching new, prolonged peak experiences of joy.

Support Groups

Finding and using a support group will serve you in many ways: emotional support, feedback from trusted others about how you are perceived, opportunity to express your emotions, self-awareness, a chance to try new ways of relating to others, learning from the lives of others, and a feeling of fulfillment in giving. Many types of groups are available in most communities, and it may take a little searching to find the one that best meets your needs. In addition to the usual clubs for overweight people, it is worth your time to check out encounter groups, sensitivity groups, integrity groups, self-development groups, etc.

Each group is different, and each group leader is different. In selecting a group that is right for you, it is important to take your time and check out two or three groups to find out what you need to know to make a good choice. Use the following criteria in evaluating a group:

1. What are the leader's credentials, training, experience, and references?
2. What is the composition of the group — how many members are there and what are their concerns? Meet the group, if possible.
3. What is the task or purpose of the group?
4. How long is the expected commitment to the group?
5. What is the fee?
6. In what type of activities will you be expected to participate?
7. What is the general philosophy on which the group is based?
8. Are the facilities adequate and appropriate?

My past research indicates that those who attended group sessions most consistently were also those who made the best weight adjustments. The group need not be specifically designed for overweight people to be effective. Some people may feel more comfortable in an overweight group; however, you aren't looking mainly for comfort, but rather a challenge and opportunity to make changes in yourself and your attitudes.

How A Group Session Works and How To Get the Most Out of It

In groups I conduct at John C. Lincoln Hospital and Health Center, Department of Health Promotions, in Phoenix, Arizona, each person in the *Total Life Weight Loss Program* is given the following guidelines:

Getting the Most Out of Group

People who *choose* to utilize group as a part of their program may find it a tremendous learning/growing experience, or a disappointing and impractical waste of time. What determines the outcome of anyone's group experience, more than the "group" itself or the facilitator, is the attitudes and expectations each individual brings to the group.

The following outline defines the group, explains how group works (its theoretical base), and how you can get the most out of it. If, after reading these guidelines, you feel that group is not for you now or in the future, you should talk to the group facilitator privately and reassess your activities in this program or explore the possibility that other programs may be more suitable for you.

The Way Group is Intended to Function

1. Group provides a special situation for ten or fewer people to develop a sharing, trusting, open atmosphere in which each individual may learn and grow along with the other group members. It is a place to deal with fears and feelings of inadequacy; to clarify values; to establish new directions and lifestyles; to discover potentials and self-identity; to build self-worth and new confidence; to realize your freedom to deal with your emotions; and to accept responsibility for your life and who you are as a person.

2. Group serves as an unstructured experience in which members determine the directions, depth, and degree of personal involvement in each session (open to all possible topics).

3. The group, by consensus, is in charge of itself. The facilitator, in the absence of group input, will offer topics, ideas, and activities, until such time as individuals or the group determines other interests and needs.

4. The time available is limited to two hours per session, per week, with an additional one-half hour, if needed, to conclude each session's discussion or activity.

5. Should an individual feel an urgent need for continued discussion following group, he or she should inform the facilitator after group session.

6. Prior to *choosing* to enter group, each person is asked to make a three-month commitment to all other group members to attend their group once each week except in the event of illness or emergency. Consistency in attendance is most important to success. However, each person is free to quit or leave group at any time. It is hoped that a decision to drop out of group would not be made without discussing it with the group as a whole, and/or the facilitator.

7. Group is intended to serve as *part* of a larger personalized program, coordinated with program counselors.

8. Group can serve as part of a larger support system by interacting, empathizing, understanding, and accepting group members who may have different circumstances from each other, but who are all attempting to make potentially stress-producing adjustments and changes.

9. Group can serve as a forum to discuss and learn of new ideas and behaviors that group members may add or drop from their lives.

10. Group can be a means of getting clear and possibly more objective feedback of how others see you, and to offer your feedback to others.

11. Group can be a safe place to try out different or new ways of interacting with people without fear of ridicule or loss of acceptance. Group can be a safe place to allow your defenses to be down and to be confronted without fear of repercussions in your family or work life.

12. Group can be a place to become more self-aware, illuminating more options to change in ways you can like yourself better. (What is "better" for you is always *your* decision.)

13. Group discussions, information, and activities hold little value until they are personalized by the individual member to see what relevance they may have in his life; therefore, a person seeking self-change has a better chance of utilizing group.

14. Group is for people who wish to change themselves as persons. Much of the desired change is found where a person has sensitive buttons touched. Human development is, therefore, often uncomfortable or painful. Emotions once feared can now be acknowledged, dealt with, and resolved if you are *willing* and *wanting* to grow. When this is so, group becomes a freeing experience that makes the discomfort all worthwhile.

Your Opportunity and Responsibility to Benefit From Group

* Be there! *Especially* if you don't feel like attending.
* Be as open and as positive to the group experience as you can.
* Encourage the quiet members to contribute and supportively confront the talkers to listen more.
* Share your opinions and feelings in balance with others.
* Remember, you can learn something of value from everyone.
* When you have strong feelings or emotions, tell the whole group *at the time* you feel them.
* When you are unhappy, dissatisfied, or angry with the direction, topic, or attitudes of the group or its members, including the facilitator, let them know *at the time,* rather than leave the group and complain to friends.
* Stay in the present and the interaction of the group. Long rambling stories are best summed up quickly in abstract form, making your points clear.
* Respect everyone's confidentiality. Leave all names and identities in the group, as you may wish to have others do with yours.
* Think of yourself as important to the group and as responsible for what happens in the group as any other member, because you are.
* Feel free to offer either controversy or agitation. Both stimulate thought, evaluation, and discussion making, which is what a group thrives on.
* Ask — don't attack. Physical attack is not permitted, and verbal attack is of little value. Honest, open questions are most valuable.
* If you have an idea, share it. New ideas, suggestions, and activities are most welcome.

* Accept new group members as opportunities, and wish the best to old members who leave.

Individual Counseling

Individuals and families all have their unique and special concerns with direct connections to the existing obesity. Not only do all of us have many concerns in common, but we also have unique bodies and minds which are influenced by obesity. With this in mind, the need for individual counseling becomes clearer. No single program, theory, or schedule is right for everybody. Objective, clear, insightful feedback is necessary to periodic adjustments (which seldom has been available within existing resources without self-promotion).

It may be beneficial to employ some type of professional counselor or psychologist to give feedback at the start of your program, with analysis of the dynamics of your weight problem, confrontation with hard-to-see blind spots, emotional support, and practical suggestions for development. Then, once a month, or every three months, use the counselor for reassessment of your whole effort. It may be that more intensive counseling could be useful until deeply ingrained problems of interpersonal communication, sexuality, emotionality, children, career, education, and social needs are relieved to make a successful focus on holistic development and permanent weight loss possible.

It is important that the proper person is utilized for professional counseling, and again, as when choosing a support group, some shopping around is advisable. Choose a counselor who meets your needs and the following criteria:

* The counselor has adequate credentials of academic training, supervised learning, and sufficient references of experience.
* The counselor has a knowledge of, and freedom from, obesity in his or her own life.

* The counselor believes in a humanistic holistic approach and clearly models that behavior in his or her own life.
* The counselor is within a reasonable distance of where you live or work, and is available for emergencies.
* The counselor's services are reasonable according to your ability to pay. If your health insurance covers psychological services, be sure the counselor is eligible to collect them.
* The counselor has a proven track record that you can easily check on with other clients and professionals who are knowledgable.
* The counselor is able to clearly describe his or her philosophy, techniques, and approach in a manner that is acceptable to you.
* The counseling facilities are comfortable and adequate to meet your needs.
* The counselor has enough breadth and depth of background that most of your various needs can be handled without bringing in other professionals.
* The counselor is a person you really respect and feel comfortable with — someone you are willing to be confronted by, and in whom you trust enough to confide your most personal feelings, thoughts, and behavior.

Existential Choices and Beliefs

The ways to development are many, and the parts of your program not specifically geared to weight loss will contribute greatly to appropriate changes. Remember, all things are connected — reading, physical development, communication skills, relaxation techniques, improved nutrition, weight loss, cosmetic improvement, self-awareness, sexuality, eliminating old fears, and so on. You may even want to take some classes or seek counseling until you develop a learning mode.

With each change you make in yourself, you'll notice your focus turns more *away* from fat and *toward* the new goals and challenges with which you are now dealing, most of which concern inappropriate eating.

In Chapter 12, reward and punishment systems are compared. If you believe a system of rewards and punishments could be useful to you in extinguishing old habits and developing new ones, then by all means employ them to your advantage. As long as *you* are clearly the decision maker, with full awareness of the conditioning process being used, any resulting credit will be yours. If you are going to incorporate behavioral methods extensively, a qualified professional should assist you.

In this Chapter, I have talked about resources, group support, family support, living and lifestyle circumstances. All these can be part of an expanded support system. Anything that provides meaning, purpose, positive reinforcement, a sense of sharing, human caring and responsibility, can be a part of a useful, growing support system. Those people who have only one or two things in their lives they care about are in a precarious emotional position, usually insecure and anxious. Those whose lives rest on many supports of interest, value, and meaning can lose one or two unexpectedly without crashing to the depths of despair and depression and becoming self-defeating in their behavior (i.e., overeating). You can expand your support system to the larger community by being part of a cause and knowing that you are contributing to others directly or indirectly by being attached to something bigger than yourself that will continue after you are gone. An idea or philosophy in which you believe can be supportive, as it will be there for you no matter what else you lose from your life. I am attached in this way to the holistic health movement and concept, and it has given me back in strength much more than I have put into it in time and effort. Build your support system whenever you can, and you will build yourself.

This is the time to start gradually determining, clarifying, and developing both your philosophy of life and the value structure upon which it rests. Every day of your life, you make hundreds of decisions which *reflect* your philosophy of life; yet if I were to ask you to *define* your philosophy of life clearly, succinctly, and completely, like most people, you would probably be at a loss. If I were to ask you to give me, in order of rank, your top ten priorities, you would probably be stuck after the first two or three.

The reason I am bringing up this lack of self-awareness is because it influences all of your behavior, emotions, and decisions to change. The unknown is upsetting, and when you don't clarify your values and philosophy of life, you do not recognize the source of your anxiety. If you have a clear, conscious awareness of your values, priorities, and philosophy of life, you are less apt to choose priority number ten over priority number two. Also, an awareness of your philosophy of life helps you to see how it contributes to your effectiveness in your day-to-day life, and this awareness enables you to like yourself for who you are.

Getting your philosophy of life and value structure clear is not done in one day. It requires a great deal of introspective thought, feedback from others, and unlimited self-observation of what you are doing, thinking, and feeling, then taking many inventories over a long period of time. It may be that it is impossible to ever be totally aware of your values and philosophy of life at any moment because you are constantly changing; but you can begin to be more aware of the questions — and the answers — and thus relieve yourself of a great deal of anxiety. It will be easier to establish clear, more meaningful directions which allow for continuing beneficial self-adjustment.

Accepting your existential choices, as defined in Chapter 11, must be continual if your self-developed program is to work for you. Determining your philosophy of life and your value structure brings this point home.

> **All it really means is that as long as you are conscious, you cannot avoid decisions.**

Accepting this idea can be your burden and fear or your freedom and adventure in life, depending upon how you choose to see it. If you choose the latter, I am sure you'll realize that the magic you were looking for outside yourself has been on the inside of you all along.

Following through on your program over a prolonged period of time means *your focus is now on what you can become.* Your motion in *becoming* is referred to as *self-actualizing.* In the process of self-actualizing, you will have moments of "peak" experience (according to Abraham Maslow's theories) when you transcend yourself — times when you reach a parallel awareness which allows you to exceed your usual limits; times when your functioning is flawless and you realize what you do is relaxed and in harmony with everything around you; intuitive moments of awareness beyond your usual capabilities.

The more self-actualizing your motion, the more often the peak experiences will occur. When you reach these experiences, fat is no longer a problem or something to fear. Overeating holds no special interest or concern for you. It is just something you are aware of in your past. You need not be or think of yourself as being handicapped again.

The point of this chapter is to lay out some possibilities from which to choose so that you might develop your own program — a program that is complete and right for you. *You can give yourself credit for what you accomplish by realizing that in the end, it is up to you to discover and bring out your own magic.*

Education

With time, experience, and continual change in yourself and all that is around you, the need for adjustment is constant. Life is continual discovery.

Even if you attempt to narrow your learning to just obesity-related data, the need for continuing education is still present. This may sound depressing if you only think of learning in the traditional sense. If you think of learning being accomplished in many ways, in many settings, and realize the doors of potential it can open, it becomes exciting. I am asking you to consider assessing your educational background in self-awareness, nutrition, exercise, psychological techniques, and humanistic existentialism, and then to make a place for future education in your new program by including one or several of the following items.

1. Reading materials (these should be used continuously).
2. Filmstrips, video and audio tapes.
3. Workshops, seminars, conferences.
4. Classes on and off campus.
5. Tutoring and apprenticeship training.
6. Personal research projects.
7. In-depth discussions with respected people.

I suggest that you also use people, gimmicks, and situations as your resources and take the overall responsibility for bringing them together; that you focus more on what you can become and less on remedial fat treatment; that you get your whole act together and not just your weight down; that if you cheat, get lazy, or permit depression, you choose to recognize it and change it — no longer waiting for someone or something to change it for you.

> **You can expect your program to be diffi-cult, to involve some expense, to be time consuming and energy draining — and that's why it will work. If you go through it all, you'll be a new person, not just a temporarily slim person.**

Remember, any good weight program will encourage you to lose slowly. One to two pounds a week is considered ideal. If you lose slowly, it is much easier on your body, and you have time to make the necessary behavioral, psychologi-cal, and attitude changes. Your practice of a lifestyle has time to become a habit and something you prefer.

From my observations, a minimum of four months is necessary to get over the attitude barriers, depending upon the degree of the weight problem; six months to a year or two is probably more realistic. This doesn't mean that all your efforts stop there. Your changes are meant for a lifetime. These are only periods when the changes in your thinking and attitude may be strengthened to the point where it is no longer a struggle.

The size of this task of bringing it all together may seem discouraging; however it takes on a snowball effect, going faster, easier, and with more momentum as it develops. *Planning for Wellness,* by Donald B. Ardell and Mark Tager, (Kendall/Hunt Publishing Co., Dubuque, Iowa), can be an excellent organizational guide for your whole effort. All the necessary charts and graphs are in a logical sequence for those of you who seek a greater degree of structure than I provide in this book. Remember though, part of the philosophy here is to seek self-awareness and spontaneity in the way you live your life and make your choices — to be the assured person who acts on life, and not simply a follower who only responds.

You know you're ready to start when:

1. You'll make time.
2. You'll give your program a very high value priority.
3. You want to change your mind as much as you want to change the weight of your body.

Briefly again, this chapter is a synthesis of all the parts of your holistic health/wellness, and taking active, practical steps to that end. Remember, the basic parts include:

* Physical fitness
* Balanced, healthful nutrition
* Stress management
* Psychological/mental health/self-awareness

and self-responsibility for all of it. In other words, to be all that you can be.

19

Staying Trim on the Road and in Spite of Those Special Occasions

During times of travel and on certain special occasions, it seems to become more difficult to maintain a healthy lifestyle. I often hear the following excuses and rationalizations for overeating and failing to exercise:

* "This will just be for a short time."
* "We've been driving all day long; I just want to stay put!"
* "I'm so tired, can't we just eat here in the hotel?"
* "Uncle Harry only comes once a year."
* "Everybody is having such a good time, why spoil it?"
* "Exercise after all that flying — are you crazy!?"
* "Let's just forget our routine for a few days, have some fun, and we'll start again when we get home."
* "My sister doesn't get married every day!"
* "Relax, it's Christmas."

There are so many times when it just seems to make sense to forget about those weeks and months of effort to get in shape and let it all hang out.

It doesn't take a week-long trip on the Orient Express to find a reason to give up healthful routines. Almost any event can qualify as a special "let's make an exception" occasion. One client even went so far as to schedule her mid-Christmas-New Year's party on the night of her support group meeting and invite all the other group members and me to attend! She honestly had not thought about the inappropriateness of this food and drink extravaganza — after all it was the holiday season.

I'm not telling you to avoid special occasions or advising you to be rigid and compulsive without allowing for fun and relaxation. What I am suggesting is that it is possible to have more energy, adventure, and pleasure on trips or at parties than ever before and arrive home feeling refreshed and rested instead of exhausted and heavy with fat and guilt.

We are beginning to realize that most of our celebrations have lost their original purpose and meaning. Celebrations intended for observing Christmas, New Years, Thanksgiving, Easter, Independence Day, anniversaries, weddings, birthdays, etc., often turn into food and drinking binges that end up leaving us disappointed in ourselves. Vacation trips and special occasions seem to be times when we abuse ourselves rather than revitalizing ourselves and rejoicing and renewing our sense of purpose and well being.

Sometimes how much you are straining and forcing yourself to do exercise and follow a healthy lifestyle, instead of learning how to change your attitudes and values, becomes clear during those special occasions or on trips. To me, special events and trips are times when my interest in healthful diet and exercise are stimulated and enhanced, not a time of "freedom" from a restrictive routine.

Having parties and house guests, for example, are times when you can show that you care about others. It is an opportunity to be creative and adventurous, not just routine. Most of all, it is your opportunity to present yourself and your values, instead of always doing what you believe to be expected of you. This may seem frightening. You don't want to jeopardize a relationship you value, yet there is much to be gained in taking the chance. You may discover which relationships are truly valuable. You could find that some relationships aren't worth maintaining if you can't be yourself. If a relationship becomes less intense, or even if it is ended, you now have room for new, more valid alliances — true kinships — that will fit into your self-development program better.

At one time, I had friends who drank alcohol, ate junk food, and smoked cigarettes. When they were guests in my home, I would try to be a good host and accommodate their lifestyle preferences, often at the expense of my own comfort. Although I still make an effort to make my friends and guests comfortable in my home, my efforts are in keeping with my own values as well as respect for their well being and health. Now my guests are offered an unpolluted environment with clean air, water, and uncontaminated healthful food, and I encourage them to participate in my own healthful lifestyle routines.

Of course when I eat in restaurants or visit a friend's house, the adjustment is for me to make, but often it becomes a compromise. At the time I accept an invitation, we discuss possibilities, and usually come to some mutually acceptable agreement ahead of time. It is not necessary to make an issue out of most arrangements, because they are usually short-term experiences. Sometimes I will eat before or after a meeting, and there are occasions that I will simply miss a meal or just drink mineral water or fruit juice. If I stay a few days with friends, I will bring certain foods along, and help with their preparation. I make sure ahead of time that my sleep and exercise routines do not disturb or interfere with my host's schedules.

Maintaining your routine while traveling can be a little more involved, and must vary with the type of transportation and locations being visited. When you travel by car, you can pack a large ice chest with things you normally eat or that might be difficult to find on the road. Having readily-available fresh fruit; vegetables such as carrots, celery, and lettuce; whole grain breads; perhaps boiled eggs and tuna; fresh fruit juices; and mineral water, etc. is an excellent way to avoid ending up at mealtime with only junk-food options. Along the way it is possible to pick up fresh items at regular grocery stores, and once you've reached a destination, with a little investigating you will usually find health food stores and natural food restaurants. Many exercises can be done in a hotel room, or a quick check with hotel personnel will let you know where it is safe to run or where there are nearby exercise facilities for whatever kind of exercise you do. Traveling by cruise ship, plane, bus, or train presents some new challenges (although some ships and airports have exercise facilities) as can staying in college dorms or in self-contained camping units — but adjustments can be made with a little forethought and some imagination.

In my personal exercise program, I use a balance of stretching, aerobic, and contractual exercises. I use weights or resistance for contractual exercising, and this sometimes presented a problem on road trips until I found the *Lifeline Gym,* a little two-pound portable gym on which I can do almost all of the muscle exercises I would normally do in a *Nautilus* spa.

Because of my eating and exercise habits, I do take a little teasing from friends and relatives at times, but I also get a whole lot of respect for living up to my convictions. You'll find that after a little thought, most people will be back to eat more of your healthful food, and they'll thank you for introducing them to it. Whether you're the guest or the host, you'll be much more interesting, and people will remember their time with you as a time when they felt good, were adventurous, interested, and felt cared about. You probably won't miss those few who don't see things that way, since they are going in a different direction than you are, pursuing a different quality of life.

> **Whatever you do, or wherever you go, you'll feel better and enjoy it more if you maintain your healthful routine.**

If you run, for example, you will see new places in a way that is much different than the view you get from a car or plane window. Finding different places to buy food can add adventure, as well as save money. Everything seems to get better and be more fun when you feel better.

These changes in lifestyle may seem a little scary, or just too complicated, and at first they do require some adjustments, but the rewards and feelings that go with your new lifestyle are hard to beat.

20

WOW I'M THIN – NOW WHAT?

CELEBRATE! CONGRATULATE YOURSELF!
Give yourself credit for what you've done and what you are
doing. Knowing that you have accepted your own freedom,
designed your own program, and most of all that you did the
work that brought you success should be a source of strength
and pride. You can call on the memory of that hard work
and the difficulties you went through to be a source of
strength when the going gets tough. You've learned to
believe in yourself for today. You have started a new lifestyle
with new attitudes and new values. The experience can
always bring you strength and hope. If you keep going, it will
bring you pleasure.

If "celebrating" means going back to your old ways or
becoming arrogant with overconfidence, you've learned very
little. But, I'm sure you realize that your achievement of
thinness is an "omega point," a way station where you like
yourself more because of the effort you are making than
because of the achievement of the goal. Luckily there is no
limit to your potential and growth, but if your effort ceases,
so will your sense of self worth. You don't go on being self-
fulfilled because you graduated from high school. The pride
of accomplishment remains, but it does not sustain you
forever.

YOU'VE LEARNED A LOT

Hopefully you have lost those unwanted pounds slowly
— not with a crash diet but rather in a way that has

expanded your self-awareness at the same time it has decreased your waistline. More awareness will always mean more options, more potentials to pursue. The effort to pursue more potential always ends up in greater personal growth.

If you were a procrastinator, hopefully you have learned to recognize the trait, to understand *why* you have procrastinated in the past, and have become willing to confront the fears or other reasons for procrastination so that you can let go of this inhibiting habit and avoid it in the future. At the same time you let go of procrastination, you had the opportunity to learn how to develop self-motivation so that you will not need Richard Simmons, or me, or magic ever again. Now you can commit yourself to the new goals you've decided upon without doubt of your willingness **and capability** to follow through. If you've come to accept the inevitability of change and your freedom to direct much of your change, you will have dealt with the fears that kept you from change in the past so that you can more easily seek new changes in the future.

If you have learned these basics in the process of losing those extra pounds, you have come a long way toward knowing how to handle the future. Whether you are dealing with love relationships, careers, diets, the environment, or the kind of person you want to be, the process is much the same. You are always seeking balance, wholeness, inner peace, and fulfillment — *"self-actualization."* You will never know total perfection, no matter how many peak experiences you may have. You'll always have the joy of something more to work for long after the memory of being fat has faded. Losing the pounds was an adventure, and if you have enough adventures, your life will be rich with quality and substance.

The idea that you always have more to do, another place to go, may sound overwhelming — like there will never be any rest, ever. However, rest is part of your new balanced lifestyle, and if you have learned how to rest well, at will, you have achieved another goal. Rest is part of a whole, and you do it over and over in between doing other things. Also, when you grow as a person, so does your energy to do more — and you need less rest. The adventure of challenge and change is exciting energy.

A NEW CHALLENGE

Being thin does carry with it some new challenges. "How do I stay this way?" "I have no handicap to use anymore. How will I face all the issues I've avoided in the past?" "What if I fail?" The answers are in the questions. *Your challenges are what enable you to maintain your momentum for constructive change.* If your focus is always on where you are going — not where you have been — you won't worry about getting fat again. It's your next achievement that interests you and requires your effort. Staying slim is just part of your new self-aware lifestyle. If you try to stand still too long, you will slip backwards. If you strain to stay the same, you will change in ways you won't like. Keep making decisions and moving forward with brief rests to celebrate. Life will never be perfect, but you will handle the problems well while experiencing tremendous fulfillment along the way.

Shedding the extra pounds and the self-defeating lifestyle that was contributing to them has created a void in your life. That space needs to be filled with something positive or fat (or something worse) will return. Selecting the things with which to fill that space can be simple — dealing with your selection may be hard.

Earlier in this book I spoke of your "buttons" (the feelings and fears you used to avoid when you were fat). The questions and new challenges in your life are the obvious fillers, along with the new potentials you discovered in the process of dealing with your buttons. Also, if you are human, you can expect to fall down from time to time. Parts of your new lifestyle and the self-awareness you now have will have to be relearned in new ways for new situations.

> **This is what is so wonderful — you always have something to work on and somewhere to go. It is change; it is life; it is what we are all about.**

All the words I've used throughout the book such as humanistic, holistic, existentialistic, creative, imaginative, balanced, potential, human growth, development, etc., lead toward self-actualization. But you only get there for brief moments. The peak experiences and times of self-transcendence come and go quickly. The human condition is never a permanent peak experience. You only have the option of working toward the peak experiences.

SELF-ACTUALIZATION IS CHANGE

To me, self-actualizing is a matter of choosing your direction. You are free to choose to lie down and die, or to be fat, or to make constructive choices in a positive direction. You may have limitations on your choices, but within those limitations, you *can* choose your directions — especially the way you are and how you choose to face life as you meet it. Sometimes the only choices you have are hard ones, but whatever they are, they are *yours*.

I have great confidence that if you accept this idea and continue to examine your philosophy of life carefully, establishing clear value structures, you will get what you need from life. You will have a sense of purpose, balance, and harmony in your life. You can see this at work in the lives of people who seem to have been given nothing, yet are more serene and at peace with themselves than those who (apparently) have everything.

The direction of self-actualizing does not appear to have an exact course (i.e., up or down); it goes where you give meaning, purpose, and feeling; where you combine body, mind, and spirit; where you are whole and in harmony with all that is around you. Only you can learn to sense where this is at any given time in your life. Only you can think your thoughts, act out your behavior, or feel your feelings. You are alone, and yet together with everything at the same time.

NOTICE: I have not given you any exact detailed instructions about personal self-actualization. The search belongs to you. It is your *freedom*. Deciding in time if what I have stated is true, is up to you. I believe you have imagination and creativity. Do you?

The theory and principles of this book are simple and old. It is the *application* of the principles which presents the problems, challenges, and questions. The more you study the existential philosophy and principles, the more you *realize* it at a non-intellectual, level. The more you feel and sense it (after accepting the logic of it), the more you realize how to apply it to your life. You realize you are very much a part of all things, and yet always an independent decision maker at the same time. As you apply what you've learned to many aspects of your life, your peace and excitement grow together. The whole process becomes as simple and clear as it was vague and confusing at the start.

One evening years ago, I watched a TV talk show that was conducted in an unusual manner. The host welcomed all his guests for the evening at the start of the show, pointing out that each person was a recognized authority in a different occupational discipline: a lawyer, a minister, an artist, an educator. The distinguished group had one question as their topic for the hour-long show: "Why are humans so inhumane to one another?" As the discussion began, each authority spoke carefully, while the others quietly awaited their turns. As the discussion progressed, voices rose, interruptions and insults were heard as they all attempted to talk at once in loud and hostile tones. The lawyer knew what we needed were more and better laws; the minister knew we needed to turn to God; the artist said we needed more beauty in our world; and, of course, the educator knew we needed more and better educational systems. Each so-called authority was intently focused upon convincing the others of the rightness of his own ideas. By the end of the program, the host had lost control of his show. Everybody was yelling and shaking fists at each other. Chaos had set in. Man's inhumanity to man was ironically visible, even as he searched for the answer as to why. When the show ended nobody was aware enough to acknowledge what had happened.

What this indicated to me was that all of the authorities had the *answer* before they started, and thus the question was never really examined. Is *knowing* the problem? If we just had the question and not the answer, would we, perhaps, have a chance? When we have a question to which we are honestly seeking an answer, our defenses are down, and we are open to learning, discovering, and changing, which is what life seems to be all about. When we have answers based on yesterday, we are unlikely to meet the new needs of today and tomorrow. Our minds are closed to new input. As long as we sincerely have questions such as "How can I be thin?", we remain open, learning, changing, and growing. When we answer a question, solve a problem, or overcome a challenge, we experience brief joy and satisfaction, but it doesn't last; we need more. We learn that our happiness is in the question.

Holistic self-development gives direction that isn't only remedial treatment, but human potential development. Without the question, the challenge, the problem, how would we gain fulfillment? If we *need* the question, shouldn't we *value* the question? If you are obese, and it is a problem, a challenge, and a question, shouldn't you view this as a means to happiness and fulfillment? Isn't the question the answer?

This philosophy applies to most things in life. Such things as diet and exercise to lose weight may never pose a challenge for you again, but all things in your life will change, and your adjustment to them is what makes life exciting, fulfilling and, joyful, or stressful, frightening and burdensome. The choice is yours. The magic is in you.

1983 METROPOLITAN HEIGHT AND WEIGHT TABLES

MEN

Height Feet	Inches	Small Frame	Medium Frame	Large Frame
5	2	128-134	131-141	138-150
5	3	130-136	133-143	140-153
5	4	132-138	135-145	142-156
5	5	134-140	137-148	144-160
5	6	136-142	139-151	146-164
5	7	138-145	142-154	149-168
5	8	140-148	145-157	152-172
5	9	142-151	148-160	155-176
5	10	144-154	151-163	158-180
5	11	146-157	154-166	161-184
6	0	149-160	157-170	164-188
6	1	152-164	160-174	168-192
6	2	155-168	164-178	172-197
6	3	158-172	167-182	176-202
6	4	162-176	171-187	181-207

WOMEN

Height Feet	Inches	Small Frame	Medium Frame	Large Frame
4	10	102-111	109-121	118-131
4	11	103-113	111-123	120-134
5	0	104-115	113-126	122-137
5	1	106-118	115-129	125-140
5	2	108-121	118-132	128-143
5	3	111-124	121-135	131-147
5	4	114-127	124-138	134-151
5	5	117-130	127-141	137-155
5	6	120-133	130-144	140-159
5	7	123-136	133-147	143-163
5	8	126-139	136-150	146-167
5	9	129-142	139-153	149-170
5	10	132-145	142-156	152-173
5	11	135-148	145-159	155-176
6	0	138-151	148-162	158-179

Courtesy of Metropolitan Life Insurance Company

TO MAKE AN APPROXIMATION OF YOUR FRAME SIZE . . .

Extend your arm and bend the forearm upward at a 90 degree angle. Keep fingers straight and turn the inside of your wrist toward your body. If you have a caliper, use it to measure the space between the two prominent bones on *either side* of your elbow. Without a caliper, place thumb and index finger of your other hand on these two bones. Measure the space between your fingers against a ruler or tape measure. Compare it with these tables that list elbow measurements for *medium-framed* men and women. Measurements lower than those listed indicate you have a small frame. Higher measurements indicate a large frame.

Height in 1" heels Men	Elbow Breadth	Height in 1" heels Women	Elbow Breadth
5'2" - 5'3"	2½" – 2⅞"	4'10" – 4'11"	2¼" – 2½"
5'4" - 5'7"	2⅝" – 2⅞"	5'0" – 5'3"	2¼" – 2½"
5'8" – 5'11"	2¾" – 3"	5'4" – 5'7"	2⅜" – 2⅝"
6'0" – 6'3"	2¾" – 3⅛"	5'8" – 5'11"	2⅜" – 2⅝"
6'4"	2⅞" – 3¼"	6'0"	2½" – 2¾"

Courtesy of Metropolitan Life Insurance Company

WEIGHT AND MEASUREMENT RECORD

How frequently you should weigh yourself depends on how consistent you have been with diet and exercise habits. If you have high expectations of more than one or two pounds of lost weight (FAT) each week, you are apt to be disappointed if you weigh too often. If you are realistic about weight loss, you will be stimulated by a one- or two-pound loss and you will not be discouraged if water retention results in no loss, or even a gain on occasion.

Weighing once a week will work best for most people if they are consistent in their efforts. If no effort has been made, then it is important to start again. Wait at least one week after beginning a renewed effort before you weigh yourself.

It is best to take measurements at the start of your program, and with every five- to ten-pound weight loss, or every thirty days in which efforts have been consistent. Remember, new lean muscle which develops from exercise will add some weight as measurements improve.

WEIGHT AND MEASUREMENT RECORD

Name _____   Height _____

Date	Weight	Loss Gain	Arms	Bust	Waist	Hips	Thighs	Ankles	Triceps	Stomach	Calf

MEASUREMENTS   CALIPERS

COMMENTS: _____

JOURNAL FOR SELF-MANAGEMENT

In an effort to manage your urges to eat inappropriately, you should start by keeping an accurate record for one or two weeks:

1. Note the hour of the day the urge was realized.
2. Indicate the strength of the urge: mild - medium - strong.
3. Describe the situation under which the urge took place — the emotion you felt, your activity, and your thoughts.
4. How did you respond to the urge? Did you eat appropriately or inappropriately? How many calories did you eat?
5. Did you respond in some manner other than eating, such as exercising? Indicate your response.

From your journal record, note your inappropriate eating patterns. Together with a counselor, plan a system of rewards for appropriate changes in your routine.

JOURNAL FOR SELF-MANAGEMENT
(sample page)

Name _____   Dated from: _____ to _____ , 19 ____

DAY	HOUR	URGE	SITUATION- Emotion, Thoughts Activity, Environment	RESPONSE

SAMPLE CONTINGENCY CONTRACT

I, _____, do hereby agree and promise to:
　　　(protagonist)

_____

_____

_____

during the time period effective _____ to _____.
In consideration, to demonstrate the sincerity of my commitment, I agree and promise to leave on deposit with _____:
　　　(administrator)

_____

_____

_____

Further, I authorize _____
　　　　　　　　　　　　　　　　　(administrator)
to turn part or all of my deposit to _____,
my favorite charity, in the event that I fail to keep any of the agreed upon conditions during the agreed upon period. Further, the exact parts of my deposit to be forfeited for my failure to meet the contingencies are:

_____

_____

_____

_____ will immediately return the remaining parts or all of the agreed upon deposit to the named person at the end of the agreed upon time. No exceptions will be made to the above conditions other than illness or emergencies serious enough to miss work.

_____
Protagonist

_____　　　_____
Witness　　　　　　　　　　　　Administrator

This also serves as a receipt for the above-named deposit.

CONTINGENCY CONTRACT

The Contingency Contract is a behavioral technique that may be freely chosen to be used for reward and punishment as a source of external motivation. It does not take the place of intrinsic motivation, but may be used temporarily as an initial stimulus.

A method of this type will help you get started in the short-term, but won't deal with underlying causes (motivations) for your weight problem and is impractical for long-term change.

How To Utilize The Contingency Contract

1. Find a person to serve as *administrator*. The administrator should be available, objective, and consistent. The protagonist must believe in the administrator as a person who is honest, just, and dependable to meet his needs.
2. The *protagonist* is the person wishing to change and put pressure on himself to carry out the activities necessary to change.
3. The protagonist places in the hands of the administrator personal property that the protagonist would be extremely reluctant to lose. If the property can be divided into parts, it will make the contract easier to administer. Money or non-property can be used. (One couple put their wedding date up as "collateral." If the protagonist didn't live up to the contingencies of the contract, the wedding date would be moved further into the future.) One person put up her paintings, which were of great value to her, and that is the key. What is put up to be earned back must be *extremely* important to the protagonist.

4. The term of the contract is usually ten to twelve weeks.
5. The administrator checks once each week. Facing the protagonist, he simply asks if the contingencies of the contract were completed. If some of the contingencies were completed, and some were not, then part or all of the property could be forfeited, depending on the specifics of the contracted agreement.
6. If the protagonist meets all contingencies of the contract, all of his property (or non-property) is returned to him at the end of the agreed upon time period.
7. Contingencies usually include such activities as:
   Exercise routines
   Diet (quantities or types of food)
   Relaxation exercise practice
   Attending a support group
   Reading self-help literature
   Communicating with supportive partners
   Any activity that is for self-improvement
8. The agreement must be signed by the protagonist, a witness, and the administrator.
9. The administrator may find it difficult to be consistent if he is a family member or a close friend.
10. The protagonist should expect the administrator to carry out the terms of the agreement, even though he knows that it may not please the protagonist.
11. If the protagonist is dishonest about his efforts, the contract loses its value.
12. If the protagonist does not live up to his agreed upon contingencies, all or part of what has been put up to be earned back is turned over to the protagonist's favorite charity for a receipt which is given to the protagonist.

GIMMICKS THAT CAN WORK

Gimmicks can be many things to many people. They can be used for self-deception and fast magic that leads to bitter resentment, lowered self-image, and increased pounds, or they can be used wisely as part of a holistic program, facilitating your efforts in a positive way. Select as many gimmicks or tricks as you believe you can feasibly fit into your program. Give them a fair trial for a period of six weeks or more. If, after that time a particular gimmick is not working for you, select another one which seems more appropriate. Additional gimmicks or variations of those listed below can be found in newspapers, magazines, books, or through your friends and weight-loss clubs. You may even create some new ones yourself.

The main determinant for the successful use of a gimmick is the degree of your belief in it. If a gimmick is presented as the sole or primary part of a weight-loss program, however, it is likely to fall short of its promise. Any gimmick you decide to use should be given careful consideration as to its psychological and physical healthfulness. The point is to use them, *with realistic expectations,* along with your total holistic program. Drugs, unusual foods, and equipment gimmicks are not included in this list.

1. Eat from a small plate to create the illusion of larger food portions.
2. Allow yourself to eat only in one designated room with only one chair at the table.
3. Place a sign in front of your eating place reminding you to eat slowly.
4. Attach an unattractive picture of yourself at your heaviest to the front of your refrigerator door.
5. Place a mirror in front of yourself when you eat and watch yourself chew.

6. After each bite of food you take, place your eating utensil on the table and place your hands in your lap while you chew.
7. Chew each bite of food a minimum of thirty times.
8. Restrict yourself to a limited number of bites per meal, regardless of which foods you eat, as long as some bites are taken from each part of a balanced menu.
9. Do a full circle observation of your nude body each morning in a full-length mirror and make a commitment to work on changing your body. Visualize how you will look when you're thin.
10. Do sixty seconds of vigorous exercise, such as running in place, before eating a meal or a midday snack.
11. Imagine your mouth being wired shut each time you have an urge to eat an inappropriate food.
12. As often as possible, substitute sexual stimulation for food when you have an urge to eat inappropriately.
13. Drink 12 ounces of water straight down before any meal or acting on an urge to snack. (This is sometimes hard on the digestion)
14. Chew low-calorie vegetables when you feel an urge to eat.
15. Do deep-breathing exercises whenever you feel an urge to eat — deeply, slowly, without straining.
16. Give yourself a non-food reward whenever you pass up an inappropriate food.
17. Take at least twenty minutes to eat a meal.
18. Buy new, attractive clothing you will be able to fit into when you have lost your unwanted pounds.
19. Tell as many people as are interested how much you weigh, that you are committed to a holistic program to get down to your ideal weight, and that you will keep them posted on your progress.

20. Place a red rubberband on your wrist and snap yourself each time you have an urge to eat inappropriately.
21. Whenever you have an urge to eat inappropriately, get a negative mental image of yourself puffing and bursting out of your best clothes.
22. Get a positive image of yourself running on the beach looking tan and lean each time you resist eating something you shouldn't.
23. Call a helping partner whenever you have an urge to go off your program and talk until the urge has passed.
24. Always park your car at least one block away from your destination and jog or walk briskly to the entrance.
25. Place a weight-loss chart or graph where you'll see it every day and weigh yourself regularly (as often as is helpful).
26. Keep a diet diary and write down your feelings, attitudes, values, successes, and commitments daily.
27. Don't take elevators or escalators. Walk or run up all stairs.
28. Analyze the food you taste for several minutes to determine if it is sour, bitter, sweet, salty, or a combination. Samples should be less than one-half teaspoon.
29. When you have an urge to eat inappropriately, stare at the food items intently for five or ten minutes and make no effort to make anything happen, or think anything, and see what occurs.
30. Use a timer when you have the urge to eat inappropriately. Set it for five minutes. Do not strain to think of anything or to keep from eating during those five minutes, and see how you feel when the time is up. (You may find it useful to extend the time later.)

31. If you have a compulsion to eat as a result of a simple oral need, substitute an infant's pacifier and use it in front of a mirror.

32. Eat with your eyes closed. See yourself getting fatter with each bite. Realize how important seeing food is to wanting food.

33. Empty your cupboards of all inappropriate and unnecessary food, then make a party or ceremony out of destroying it as you make your commitment to a new healthy life.

34. When you have an urge to eat inappropriately, stimulate your non-taste senses through an activity such as smelling flowers.

35. If your hunger is the result of emotions and you are using food to soothe your feelings, reach out and get a hug from the closest person, or call someone you love and tell them you love them.

FIFTY EXCUSES
FOR STAYING FAT
OR GETTING FATTER

If you wish to weaken your self-image and resolve, here are fifty common reasons for going off your program. You may want to add your own favorite excuses to this list and then let them go from your thought and speech habits. Remember, if you should fall down in your effort to be consistent, it is important to forgive yourself and to re-establish your resolve to reach your goal.

1. It rained today.
2. I felt depressed.
3. We had company.
4. I was tired from work.
5. I've just been too busy lately.
6. I don't feel well.
7. It's too cold (or too hot).
8. I get bored.
9. My partner couldn't go today.
10. My muscles hurt.
11. It's too late (early) now.
12. It's such hard work.
13. It's not safe to run around here.
14. I have no energy.
15. I need to be with a group.
16. I have no place to do it.
17. I couldn't do it during the holidays.
18. I don't lose weight when I exercise or diet anyway.
19. I have a headache.
20. Nobody will do it with me.
21. It's dark when I get up.

22. I forgot.
23. It didn't change my body anyway.
24. My kids needed me.
25. I don't have time.
26. I read an article that said dieting and exercising aren't good for you.
27. My doctor said if I run my uterus will fall.
28. I know a person who never diets or exercises, and she's in great shape.
29. Why get in shape? I'll just get out of shape again, anyway.
30. It costs too much.
31. I don't want to develop masculine-looking muscles.
32. Uncle Harry doesn't like to eat or drink alone.
33. It was such a special occasion.
34. I couldn't just waste it or throw it out.
35. Everybody else had some and I didn't want to be a party pooper.
36. My kids would really be unhappy if we didn't have sweets in the house.
37. It was like Jack-In-the-Box was calling me.
38. I have to taste what I cook.
39. One little piece won't hurt.
40. I exercised extra hard today and I deserve this little treat.
41. It is the only thing that calms me down.
42. I didn't read the label.
43. I was so preoccupied, I just didn't notice what I was eating.
44. I may never have the chance again.
45. I just knew it would be the last time.
46. I was mad and didn't care anymore.
47. It was junk food or nothing.
48. I had been dreaming about it for a week.

49. I wanted to get back at him.
50. But I've lost twenty pounds.
51. _____
52. _____
53. _____
54. _____
55. _____

FOOD COMPOSITION

100 grams, edible portion

(dash (—) denotes lack of reliable data for a constituent believed to be present in measurable amount)

FOOD	CALORIES	PROTEINS grams	FATS grams	CARBOHYDRATES grams	CALCIUM mg.	PHOSPHORUS mg.	MAGNESIUM mg.	IRON mg.	SODIUM mg.	POTASSIUM mg.	VITAMIN A VALUE IU	B_1 mg.	B_2 mg.	NIACIN mg.	VITAMIN C mg.
ACEROLA cherry, raw	28	.4	.3	6.8	12	11	—	.2	8	83	—	.02	.06	0.4	1,300
ACEROLA JUICE, raw	23	.4	.3	4.8	10	9	—	.5	3	—	—	.02	.06	.4	1,600
ALMONDS, dried	598	18.6	54.2	19.5	234	504	270	4.7	4	773	0	.24	.92	3.5	trace
APPLES, freshly harvested	58	.2	.6	14.5	7	10	8	.3	1	110	90	.03	.02	.4	7-20
APPLE JUICE, canned or bottled	47	.1	trace	11.9	6	9	4	.6	1	101	—	.01	.02	.1	1
APRICOTS, raw	51	1.0	.2	12.8	17	23	12	.5	1	281	2,700	0.3	.04	.6	10
APRICOTS, dried, uncooked	260	5.0	.5	66.5	67	108	62	5.5	26	979	10,900	.01	.16	3.3	12
ARTICHOKES, globe or French, raw	9-47	2.9	0.2	10.6	51	88	—	1.3	43	430	160	.01	.05	1.0	12
cooked	8-44	2.8	.2	9.6	51	68	—	1.1	30	301	150	.08	.04	.7	8
ARTICHOKES, Jerusalem, raw	7-75	2.3	.1	16.7	14	78	11	3.4	—	—	20	.07	.06	1.3	4
ASPARAGUS, raw spears	26	2.5	.2	5.0	22	62	20	1.0	2	278	900	.2	.20	1.5	33
cooked spears	20	2.2	.2	3.6	21	50	14	.6	1	183	900	.18	.18	1.4	26
AVOCADOS, raw	167	2.1	16.4	6.3	10	42	45	.6	4	604	290	.16	.20	1.6	14
BANANAS, common, raw	85	1.1	.2	22.2	8	26	33	.7	1	370	190	.11	.06	.7	10
BARLEY, pearled, light	349	8.2	1.0	78.8	16	189	37	2.0	3	160	0	.12	.05	3.1	0

BEANS, common white, cooked	118	7.8	.6	21.2	50	148	37	2.7	7	416	0	.14	.07	.7	0
red, cooked	347	7.8	.5	21.4	38	140		2.7	3	340	trace	.11	.06	.7	
pinto, raw	349	22.9	1.2	63.7	135	457		6.4	10	984		.84	.21	2.2	29
lima, immature cooked	123	8.4	.5	22.1	52	142	46	2.8	2	650	290	.24	.12	1.4	
lima, mature, cooked	138	8.2	.6	25.6	29	154	48	3.1	2	612	20	.13	.06	.7	19
mung, sprouted, raw	38	3.8	.2	6.6	19	64		1.3	5	223	600	.13	.13	.8	19
green, raw	32	1.9	.2	7.1	56	44	32	.8	7	243	540	.8	.11	.5	12
green, cooked	25	1.6	.2	5.4	50	37	21	.6	4	151	20	.07	.09	.5	10
BEETS, red, raw	43	1.6	.1	9.9	16	33	25	.7	60	335	20	.03	.05	.4	6
red, cooked	32	1.1	.1	7.2	14	23	15	.5	43	208	20	.03	.04	.3	
BEET GREENS, raw	24	2.2	.3	4.6	119	40	106	3.3	130	570	6,100	.10	.22	.4	30
cooked	18	1.7	.2	3.3	99	25		1.9	76	332	5,000	.07	.15	.3	15
BLACKBERRIES, raw	58	1.2	.9	12.9	32	19	30	.9	1	170	200	.03	.04	.4	21
BLUEBERRIES, raw	62	.7	.5	15.3	15	13	6	1.0	1	81	100	.03	.06	.5	14
BRAZIL NUTS, raw	654	14.3	66.9	10.9	186	693	225	3.4	1	715	trace	.96	.12	1.6	
BROCCOLI, raw spears	32	3.6	.3	5.9	103	78	24	1.1	15	382	2,500	.10	.23	.9	113
cooked	26	3.1	.3	4.5	88	62	21	.8	10	267	2,500	.09	.20	.8	90
BRUSSELS SPROUTS, raw	45	4.9	.4	8.3	36	80	29	1.5	14	390	550	.10	.16	.9	102
cooked	36	4.2	.4	6.4	32	72	21	1.1	10	273	520	.08	.14	.8	87
BUCKWHEAT, whole grain	335	11.7	2.4	72.9	114	282	229	3.1		448	0	.60		4.4	0
BUTTER, salted	716	.6	81.	.4	20	16	2	0	987	23	3,300				0
unsalted	720	.6	82.	.4	20	16		0	8	9	3,350			0	
BUTTERMILK, cultured, from skim milk	36	3.6	.1	5.1	121	95	14	trace	130	140	trace	.4	.18	.1	1
CABBAGE, white, raw	24	1.3	.2	5.4	49	29	13	.4	20	233	130	.05	.05	.3	47
red, raw	31	2.0	.2	6.9	42	35		.8	26	268	40	.09	.06	.4	61
savoy, raw	24	2.4	.2	4.6	67	54		.9	22	269	200	.05	.08	.3	55
CAROB FLOUR	180	4.5	1.4	80.7	352	81							.25		
CARROTS, raw	42	1.1	.2	9.7	37	36	23	.7	47	341	11,000	.06	.05	.6	8
CASHEW NUTS	561	17.2	45.7	29.3	38	373	267	3.8	15	464	100	.43	.10	1.8	
CALIFLOWER, raw	27	2.7	.2	5.2	25	56	24	1.1	13	295	60	.11	.08	.7	78
cooked	22	2.3	.2	4.1	21	42		.7	9	206	60	.09	.03	.6	55
CELERY, raw	17	.9	.1	3.9	39	28	22	.3	126	341	240	.03	.03	.3	9
CHARD, Swiss, raw	25	2.4	0.3	4.6	88	39	65	3.2	147	550	6,500	.06	.17	.5	32
cooked	18	1.8		3.3	73	24		1.8	86	321	5,400	.04	.11	.4	16

Reprinted by permission, from VITAMINS & MINERALS — THE HEALTH CONNECTION, Health Plus Publishers.

FOOD	CALORIES	PROTEINS grams	FATS grams	CARBOHYDRATES grams	CALCIUM mg.	PHOSPHORUS mg.	MAGNESIUM mg.	IRON mg.	SODIUM mg.	POTASSIUM mg.	VITAMIN A VALUE IU	B₁ mg	B₂ mg	NIACIN mg.	VITAMIN C mg.
CHEESE, Blue or Roquefort	368	21.5	30.5	2.0	315	339	48	.5	700	82	1,240	.03	.61	1.2	
Cheddar	398	25.0	32.2	2.1	750	478	45	1.0	229	85	1,310	.03	.46	.1	
Cottage, creamed	106	13.6	4.2	2.9	94	152	—	.3	290	72	170	.03	.25	.1	
Cottage, uncreamed	86	17.0	.3	2.7	90	175	—	.4	710	104	10	.03	.28	.1	
Swiss	370	27.5	28.0	1.7	925	563	—	.9		—	1,140	.01	.40	.1	
Brick	370	22.2	30.5	1.9	730	455	—	.9		—	1,240	—	.45	.1	
CHERRIES, sour, red, raw	58	1.2	.3	14.3	29	19	14	.4	2	191	1,000	.05	.06	.4	10
sweet, raw	70	1.3	.3	17.4	22	19	9	.4	2	191	110	.05	.06	.4	10
frozen, sour, red	55	1.0	.4	13.4	13	22	10	.7	2	188	1,000	.04	.07	.3	5
CHESTNUTS, fresh	194	2.9	1.5	42.1	27	88	41	1.7	6	454	—	.22	.22	.6	
COCONUT MEAT, fresh	346	3.5	35.3	9.4	13	95	46	1.7	23	256	0	.05	.02	.5	3
dried	662	7.2	64.9	23.0	26	187	90	3.3	—	588	0	.06	.04	.6	0
COCONUT WATER, from green coconuts	22	.3	.2	4.7	20	13	28	.3	25	147	0	trace	trace	.1	2
COLLARDS, raw, leaves	45	4.8	0.8	7.5	250	82	57	1.5	—	450	9,300	0.16	.31	1.7	152
cooked	33	3.6	.7	5.1	188	52	38	.8	—	262	7,800	.11	.20	1.2	76
CORN, whole-grain, dried, raw	348	8.9	3.9	72.0	22	268	147	2.1	1	284	490	.37	.12	2.2	
SWEET, on-the-cob, raw	96	3.5	1.0	22.0	3	111	48	.7	trace	280	400	.15	.12	1.7	12
cooked on the cob	91	3.3	1.0	21.0	3	89	19	.6	trace	196	400	.12	.10	1.4	9
flour	368	7.8	2.6	76.8	6	164	106	1.8	1	—	340	.20	.06	1.4	
bread, whole-grain	207	7.4	7.2	29.1	120	211	—	1.1	628	157	150	.13	.19	.6	1
CRANBERRIES, raw	46	.4	.7	10.8	14	10	8	.5	2	82	40	.03	.02	.1	11
CUCUMBERS, raw	15	.9	.1	3.4	25	27	11	1.1	6	160	250	.03	.04	.2	11

FOOD															
CURRANTS, black, raw	54	1.7	.1	13.1	60	40	15	1.1	3	372	230	.05	.05	.3	200
DANDELION GREENS, raw	45	2.7	.7	9.2	187	66	36	3.1	76	397	14,000	.19	.26	—	35
DATES	274	2.2	.5	72.9	59	63	58	3.0	1	648	50	.09	.10	2.2	0
EGGS, whole, raw	163	12.9	11.5	.9	54	205	11	2.3	122	129	1,180	.11	.30	.1	0
yolks, raw	348	16.0	30.6	.6	141	569	16	5.5	52	98	3,400	.22	.44	.1	0
cooked, whole	163	12.9	11.5	.9	54	205		2.3	122	129	1,180	.09	.28	.1	0
EGGPLANT, cooked	19	1.0	.2	4.1	11	21		.6	1	150	10	.05	.04	.5	3
ELDERBERRIES, raw	72	2.6	.5	16.4	38	28	10	1.6	—	300	600	.07	.06	.5	36
ENDIVE, raw	20	1.7	.1	4.1	181	54	20	1.7	14	294	3,300	.07	.14	.5	10
FIGS, raw	80	1.2	.3	20.3	35	22	71	.6	2	194	80	.06	.05	.4	2
dried	274	4.3	1.3	69.1	126	77	184	3.0	34	640	80	.10	.10	.7	0
FILBERTS (hazelnuts)	634	12.6	62.4	16.7	209	337	36	3.4	2	704	—	.46	—	.9	trace
GARLIC, raw	137	6.2	.2	30.8	29	202	9	1.5	19	529	trace	.25	.08	.5	15
GOOSENBERRIES, raw	39	0.8	.2	9.7	18	15	12	0.5	1	155	290	—	—	.2	33
GRAPEFRUIT, raw	41	.5	.1	10.6	16	16	12	.4	1	135	80	.04	.02	.2	38
juice	39	.5	.1	9.2	9	15	13	.2	1	162	80	.04	.02	.2	38
GRAPES, raw	69	1.3	1.0	15.7	16	12	13	.4	3	158	100	.05	.03	.3	4
juice, bottled	66	.2	trace	16.6	11	12	13	.3	2	116	—	.04	.02	.2	trace
GUAVAS, whole, raw	62	.8	.6	15.	23	42	3	.9	4	289	280	.05	.05	1.2	242
HONEY	304	.3	0	82.3	5	6	34	.5	5	51	0	trace	.04	.3	1
HORSERADISH, raw	87	3.2	.3	19.7	140	64	37	1.4	8	564	—	.07	—	—	81
KALE, leaves, raw	53	6.0	.8	9.0	249	93	740	2.7	75	378	10,000	.17	.26	2.1	186
cooked	39	4.5	.7	6.1	187	58	37	1.6	43	221	8,300	.10	.18	1.6	93
KELP, raw		5.0	1.1		1,093	240	—	3.7	3,007	5,273	—	—	—	—	5-140
KOHLRABI, raw	29	2.0	.1	6.6	41	51	10	.5	8	372	20	.06	.04	.3	66
KUMQUATS, raw	65	.9	.1	17.1	63	23	8	.4	7	236	600	.08	.10	—	36
LEMONS, peeled, raw	27	1.1	.3	8.2	26	16	80	.6	2	138	20	.04	.02	.1	53
LEMON JUICE, raw	25	.5	.2	8.0	7	10	—	.2	1	141	20	.03	.01	.1	46
LENTILS, dry, cooked	106	7.8	trace	19.3	25	119	11	2.1	—	249	20	.07	.06	.6	0
LETTUCE, raw, romaine	18	1.3	.3	3.5	68	25	18	1.4	9	264	1,900	.05	.08	.4	18
Iceberg, New York	13	.9	.1	2.9	20	22		.5	9	175	330	.06	.06	.3	6
MANGOS, raw	66	.7	.4	16.8	10	13		.4	7	189	4,800	.05	.05	1.1	35

FOOD	CALORIES	PROTEINS grams	FATS grams	CARBOHYDRATES grams	CALCIUM mg	PHOSPHORUS mg	MAGNESIUM mg	IRON mg	SODIUM mg	POTASSIUM mg	VITAMIN A VALUE IU	B1 mg	B2 mg	NIACIN mg	VITAMIN C mg
MILK, cow's, whole	65	3.5	3.5	4.9	118	93	13	trace	50	144	140	.03	.17	.1	1
skim	36	3.6	.1	5.1	121	95	14	trace	52	145	trace	.04	.18	.1	1
dry, whole	502	26.4	27.5	38.2	909	708	98	.5	405	1,330	1,130	.29	1.46	.7	6
dry, skim non-instant	363	35.9	.8	52.3	1,308	1,016	143	.6	532	1,745	30	.35	1.80	.9	7
MILK, goat's, raw	67	3.2	4.0	4.6	129	106	17	.1	34	180	160	.04	.11	.3	1
MILLET, whole-grain	327	9.9	2.9	72.9	20	311	162	6.8		430	0	.73	.38	2.3	0
MOLASSES, blackstrap	213			55	684	84	258	16.1	96	2,927		.11	.19	2.0	
MUSHROOMS, cultivated, raw	28	2.7	.3	4.4	6	116	13	.8	15	414	trace	.10	.46	4.2	3
MUSKMELONS, raw, cantaloupe	30	.7	.1	7.5	14	16	16	.4	12	251	3,400	.04	.03	.6	33
honeydew	33	.8	.3	7.7	14	16		.4	12	251	40	.04	.03	.6	23
MUSTARD GREENS, raw	31	3.0	.5	5.6	183	50	27	3.0	32	377	7,000	.11	.22	.8	97
NECTARINES, raw	64	.6	trace	17.1	4	24	13	.5	6	294	1,650				13
OATMEAL or rolled oats, dry	390	14.2	7.2	68.2	53	405	144	4.5	2	352	0	.60	.14	1.0	0
cooked	55	2.0	1.0	9.7	9	57	21	.6		61	0	.08	.02	.1	0
OKRA, raw	36	2.4	.3	7.6	92	51	41	.6	3	249	520	.17	.21	1.0	31
ONIONS, mature, raw	38	1.5	.1	8.7	27	36	12	.5	10	157	40	.03	.04	.2	10
green, bulb & top	36	1.5	.2	8.2	51	39		1.0	5	237	2,000	.05	.05	.4	32
ORANGES, peeled, raw	49	1.0	.2	12.2	41	20	11	.4	1	200	200	.10	.04	.4	50
ORANGE JUICE, raw	45	.7	.2	10.2	11	17	11	.2	1	200	200	.09	.03	.4	50
PAPAYA, raw	39	.6	.1	10.0	20	16		.3	3	234	1,750	.04	.04	.3	56
PARSLEY, raw	44	3.6	.6	8.5	203	63	41	6.2	45	727	8,500	.12	.26	1.2	172
PARSNIPS, raw	76	1.7	.5	17.5	50	77	32	.7	12	541	30	.07	.08	.1	10
PEACHES, raw	38	.6	.1	9.7	9	19	10	.5	1	202	1,330	.02	.05	1.0	7
PEANUTS, raw, with skins	564	26.0	47.5	18.6	68	401	206	2.1	5	674		1.14	.13	17.2	0

234

Food														
PEARS, raw	61	.7	.4	15.3	8	11	7	.3	2	130	20	.02	.04	.1
PEAS, raw, from pods	53	3.4	.2	12.0	62	90	35	.7	1	170	680	.28	.12	—
green, cooked	71	5.4	.4	12.1	23	99	—	1.8	13	196	540	.28	.11	2.3
split, cooked	115	8.0	.3	20.8	11	89	—	1.7	trace	296	40	.15	.09	.9
PECANS	687	9.2	71.2	14.6	73	289	142	2.4	13	603	130	.86	.13	.9
PEPPERS, raw, sweet, green	22	1.2	.2	4.8	9	22	18	.7	trace	213	420	.08	.08	.5
raw, red	31	1.4	.3	7.1	13	30	—	.6	13	—	4,450	.08	.08	.5
PERSIMMONS, raw	127	.8	.4	33.5	27	26	8	2.5	—	310	—	—	—	—
PINEAPPLE, raw	52	0.4	0.2	13.7	17	8	13	0.5	1	146	70	.09	.03	.2
juice, canned, unsweetened	55	.4	.4	13.5	15	9	12	.3	1	149	50	.05	.02	.2
PLUMS, prune-type, raw	75	.8	.2	19.7	12	18	9	.5	1	170	300	.03	.03	.5
POTATOES, raw	76	2.1	.1	17.1	7	53	34	.6	3	407	trace	.10	.04	1.5
baked in skin	93	2.6	.1	21.1	9	65	—	.7	4	503	trace	.10	.04	1.7
boiled in skin	76	2.1	.1	17.1	7	53	—	.6	3	407	trace	.09	.04	1.5
PUMPKIN, raw	26	1.0	.1	6.5	21	44	12	.8	1	340	1,600	.05	.11	.6
PUMPKIN SEEDS, dry	553	29.0	46.7	15.0	51	1,144	—	11.2	—	—	—	.24	.19	2.4
RADISHES, raw	17	1.0	.1	3.6	30	31	15	1.0	18	322	10	.03	.03	.3
RAISINS, natural, uncooked	289	2.5	.2	77.4	62	101	35	3.5	27	763	20	.11	.08	.5
RASPBERRIES, raw, black	73	1.5	1.4	15.7	30	22	30	0.9	1	199	trace	.03	.09	0.9
red	57	1.2	.5	13.6	22	22	20	0.9	—	168	130	.03	.09	0.9
RICE, brown, cooked	119	2.5	.6	25.5	12	73	29	.5	3	70	0	.09	.02	1.4
RICE BRAN	276	13.3	15.8	50.8	76	1,386	—	19.4	trace	1,495	0	2.26	.25	29.8
RICE POLISHINGS	265	12.1	12.8	57.7	69	1,106	—	16.1	trace	714	0	1.84	.18	28.2
RUTABAGAS, raw	46	1.1	.1	11.0	66	39	15	.4	5	239	580	.07	.07	1.1
cooked	35	.9	.1	8.2	59	31	—	.3	4	167	550	.06	.06	.8
RYE, whole-grain	334	12.1	1.7	73.4	38	376	115	3.7	1	467	0	.43	.22	1.6
flour, dark	327	16.3	2.6	68.1	54	536	73	4.5	1	860	0	.61	.22	2.7
SAUERKRAUT, solids and liquid	18	1.0	.2	4.0	36	18	—	.5	—	140	50	.03	.04	.2
SESAME SEEDS, dry, whole	563	18.6	49.1	21.6	1,160	616	181	10.5	60	725	30	.98	.24	5.4
SOYBEANS, dry, raw	403	34.1	17.7	33.5	226	554	265	8.4	5	1,677	80	1.10	.31	2.2
cooked	130	11.0	5.7	10.8	73	179	—	2.7	2	540	30	.21	.09	.6
sprouted, raw	46	6.2	1.4	5.3	48	67	—	1.0	—	—	80	.23	.20	.8
sprouted, cooked	38	5.3	1.4	3.7	43	50	—	.7	—	—	80	.16	.15	.7

Last column (Ascorbic acid):
PEARS 4; PEAS 21; green 20; split —; PECANS 2; PEPPERS green 128; red 204; PERSIMMONS 66; PINEAPPLE 17; juice 9; PLUMS 4; POTATOES raw 20; baked 20; boiled 16; PUMPKIN 9; PUMPKIN SEEDS —; RADISHES 26; RAISINS 1; RASPBERRIES black 18; red 25; RICE brown 0; RICE BRAN 0; RICE POLISHINGS 0; RUTABAGAS raw 43; cooked 26; RYE whole-grain 0; flour dark 0; SAUERKRAUT 14; SESAME 0; SOYBEANS raw —; cooked 0; sprouted raw 13; sprouted cooked 4.

Food														
SOYBEAN CURD (TOFU)	72	7.8	4.2	2.4	128	126	111	1.9	7	42	0	.06	.03	.1	—
SOYBEAN FLOUR, full-fat	421	36.7	20.3	30.4	199	558	247	8.4	1	1,660	110	.85	.31	2.1	0
SOYBEAN MILK, powder	429	41.8	20.3	28.0	278		300								
SPINACH, raw	26	3.2	.3	4.3	93	51	88	3.1	71	470	8,100	.10	.20	.6	51
cooked	23	3.0	.3	3.6	93	38	65	2.2	50	324	8,000	.07	.14	.5	28
SQUASH, summer, all varieties, raw	19	1.1	.1	4.2	28	29	16	.4	1	202	410	.05	.09	1.0	22
cooked	14	.9	.1	3.1	25	25	16	.4	1	141	370	.05	.08	.8	10
winter, raw	50	1.4	.3	12.4	22	38	17	.6	1	369	3,700	.05	.11	.6	13
cooked (baked)	63	1.8	.5	15.4	28	48	17	.8	1	461	4,200	.05	.13	.7	13
STRAWBERRIES, raw	37	.7	.4	8.4	21	21	12	1.0	1	164	60	.03	.07	.6	59
SUNFLOWER SEED KERNELS, dry	560	24.0	47.3	19.9	120	837	38	7.1	30	920	50	1.96	.23	5.4	—
TOMATOES, ripe, raw	22	1.1	.2	4.7	13	27	14	.5	3	244	900	.06	.04	.7	23
TOMATO JUICE, canned	19	.9	.1	4.3	7	18	10	.9	200	227	800	.05	.03	.8	16
TURNIPS, raw	30	1.0	.2	6.6	39	30	20	.5	49	268	trace	.04	.07	.6	36
cooked	23	.8	.3	4.9	35	24	—	.4	34	188	trace	.04	.05	.3	22
TURNIP GREENS, raw	28	3.0	.3	5.0	246	58	58	1.8	—	—	7,600	.21	.39	.8	139
WALNUTS, black	628	20.5	59.3	14.8	trace	570	190	6.0	3	460	300	.22	.11	.7	—
English	651	14.8	64.0	15.8	99	380	131	3.1	2	450	30	.33	.13	.9	2
WATERCRESS, raw	19	2.2	.3	3.0	151	54	20	1.7	52	282	4,900	.08	.16	.9	79
WATERMELON, raw	26	.5	.2	6.4	7	10	8	.5	1	100	590	.03	.03	.2	7
WHEAT, whole-grain, spring	330	14.0	2.2	69.1	36	383	160	3.1	3	370	—	.57	.12	4.3	0
winter	330	12.3	1.8	71.7	46	354	160	3.4	3	370	—	.52	.12	4.3	0
WHEAT BRAN	213	16.0	4.6	61.9	119	1,276	490	14.9	9	1,121	0	.72	.35	21.0	0
WHEAT GERM, raw	363	26.6	10.9	46.7	72	1,118	336	9.4	3	827	0	2.01	.68	4.2	0
WHEY, powder	349	12.9	1.1	73.5	646	589	130	1.4	—	—	0	.50	2.51	.8	—
YAM, tuber, raw	101	2.1	.2	23.2	20	69	31	.6	—	600	50	.10	.04	.5	9
YEAST, brewer's debittered	283	38.8	1.0	38.4	210	1,753	231	17.3	121	1,894	trace	15.61	4.28	37.9	trace
torula	277	38.6	1.0	37.0	424	1,713	165	19.3	15	2,046	trace	14.01	5.06	44.4	trace
YOGURT, from whole milk	62	3.0	3.4	4.9	111	87	12	trace	47	132	140	.03	.16	.1	1
from skimmed milk	50	3.4	1.7	5.2	120	94	13	trace	51	143	70	.04	.18	.1	1

SOURCES: Agriculture Handbook No. 8., U.S. Dept. Agric. Washington, D.C.; Home and Garden Bulletin No. 72.

RECOMMENDED READING

The Airola Diet & Cookbook, Paavo Airola, Ph.D. and Anni Airola Lines, R.D., Health Plus Publishers, Phoenix, AZ, 1981.

Bulimarexia, M. B. White, Ph.D., and Wm. C. White, Ph.D., W. W. Norton & Co., Inc., New York, NY, 1983.

Excessive Eating, Joyce Ann Slochower, Ph.D., Human Sciences Press, Inc. New York, NY, 1983.

14 Days to a Wellness Lifestyle, Donald Ardell, Ph.D., Whatever Publishing, Inc., Mill Valley, CA, 1982.

How To Get Well, Paavo Airola, Ph.D., Health Plus Publishers, Phoenix, AZ 1974.

In the Mind's Eye, Arnold Lazarus, Ph.D., The Guilford Press, New York, NY, 1977.

Nutraerobics, Jeffrey Bland, Ph.D., Harper & Row, New York, NY 1983.

Overcoming Indecisiveness, Theodore Isaac Rubin, M.D., Harper & Row, New York, NY, 1985.

Planning for Wellness, Donald B. Ardell, Ph.D. and Mark J. Tager, M.D., Kendall/Hunt Publishing Co., Dubuque, IA, 1982.

Self-Watching, Roger Hodgson and Peter Miller, Facts on File, Inc., New York, NY 1982.

Sweet Suffering, Natalie Shainess, M.D., Bobbs-Merrill, Indianapolis, IN, 1984.

The Ultimate Athlete, George Leonard, Viking, New York, NY, 1975.

Vitamins & Minerals: The Health Connection, Anni Airola Lines, R.D., Health Plus Publishers, Phoenix, AZ, 1985.

Wellness Workbook, Regina Sara Ryan and John W. Travis, M.D., Ten Speed Press, Berkeley, CA, 1981.

BIBLIOGRAPHY

Abramson, E. E. and S. G. Stinson, "Boredom and Eating In Obese and Non-obese Individuals," *Addictive Behaviors,* 1977, pp. 2, 181-185.

Adler, Jerry and Mariana Gosnell, "What It Means To Be Fat," *Newsweek,* December 1982, p.84.

Akers, Keith, "Why People Get Fat," *Vegetarian Times,* May 1983, pp. 28-31.

Allen, Robert F., *Stress Reduction and Weight Control,* New York, NY: Appleton-Century-Crofts, 1981.

Anderson, Robert A., *Stress Power,* New York, NY: Human Sciences Press, 1977.

Ardell, Donald B., *14 Days To A Wellness Lifestyle,* Mill Valley, CA: Whatever Publishing, Inc., 1982.

Ardell, Donald B. and Mark J. Tager, *Planning for Wellness,* Dubuque, IA: Kendall/Hunt Publishing Co., 1982.

Bailey, Covent, *Fit or Fat,* Boston, MA: Houghton Mifflin, 1978.

Bakker, Cornelis B., "Why People Change," *Psychotherapy: Theory, Research and Practice,* Summer 1975, 12:2.

Barrow, John C. and Carol A. Moore, "Group Interventions With Perfectionist Thinking," *The Personnel & Guidance Journal,* June 1983, pp. 612-615.

Beller, Anne Scott, *Fat and Thin,* New York, NY: McGraw-Hill, 1978.

Benson, Herbert, "Harvard Professor Proves That Meditation Lowers Blood Pressure," *Holistic Health & Medicine,* December 1984, pp. 24-32.

Berger, Stuart, M., *Dr. Berger's Immune Power Diet,* New York, NY: New American Library, 1985.

Berland, Theodore, *Rating The Diets, (Consumer Guide),* Skokie, IL: Publications International, Ltd., 1974.

Bernard, J. L., "Rapid Treatment of Gross Obesity by Operant Techniques," *Psychological Reports,* 1969, pp. 23, 663-666.

Bland, Jeffrey, "The Junk Food Syndrome," *Psychology Today,* January 1982, p. 92.

Bland, Jeffrey, *Nutraerobics,* San Francisco, CA: Harper & Row, 1983.

Bland, Jeffrey, *Year Book of Nutritional Medicine,* New Canaan, CT: Keats Publishing, 1984.

Bland, Jeffrey, *Your Health Under Siege,* Brattleboro, VT: The Stephen Greene Press, 1981.

Bland, Jeffrey and Norman Shealy, *Medical Applications of Clinical Nutrition,* New Canaan, CT: Keats Publishing, 1983.

Branden, Nathaniel, *The Psychology of Romantic Love,* New York, NY: Bantam Books, 1983.

Bray, George A., Editor, *Fogerty International Center Series on Preventive Medicine, Vol. III, Part I,* National Institute of Health, Bethesda, MD: U.S. Department of Health Education and Welfare Publications #NIH-75-708, 1973.

Brennan, R.O., *Nutrigenetic,* New York, NY: Signet, 1977.

Breznitz, Shlomo, "To Dream the Possible Dream," *American Health,* December 1984, pp. 60-61.

Bruno, Frank J., *Think Yourself Thin,* New York, NY: Barnes & Noble Books, 1973.

Buckley, Marcie, "Wellness In The Workplace," *Holistic Life Magazine,* Summer 1982, pp. 6-7, 57.

Burns, David D., "The Perfectionist's Script for Self-Defeat,"

Cheraskin, E. and W. M. Ringsdorf, with Arlene Brecker, *Psychodietetics,* New York, NY: Bantam Books, 1974.

Charlesworth, Edward A. and Ronald G. Nathan, *Stress Management — A Comprehensive Guide To Wellness,* Houston, TX: Biobehavioral Press, 1982.

Choate, Robert, and Aaron and Cardillo Smith, and Joseph E. and Leslie Thompson, "Training In The Use of Goal Attainment Scaling," *Community Mental Health Journal,* Summer 1981, 17:171-181.

Cohen, William S., "Health Promotion In The Workplace," *American Psychologist,* February 1985, 40:2, pp. 213-216.

Cooper, Kenneth H., *The Aerobics Way,* New York, NY: Evans and Co., 1979.

Cotter, Sherwin B. and Julio J. Guerra, *Assertion Training,* Champaign, IL: Research Press Co., 1979.

Creekmore, C. R., "Games Athletes Play," *Psychology Today,* July 1984, pp. 40-44.

Dusek, Dorothy E., *Thin & Fit: Your Personal Lifestyle,* Belmont, CA: Wadsworth Publishing Co., 1982.

Ellis, Albert and William J. Knaus, *Overcoming Procrastination,* New York, NY: New American Library, 1977.

Facts About Obesity, National Institute of Health, Superintendent of Document, U.S. Government Printing Office, Washington, D.C.: 1977.

Ferguson, J., *Habits Not Diets,* Palo Alto, CA: Bull Publishers, 1976.

Fixx, Jim, *Second Book of Running,* New York, NY: Random House, 1980.

Food and Your Weight, Home and Garden Bulletin #74, U.S. Department of Agriculture, Washington, D.C.: 1977.

Foreyt, J. P. and W. A. Kennedy, "Treatment of Overweight by Aversion Therapy," *Behavior Research and Therapy,* 1971, pp. 9, 29-34.

Fredericks, Carlton, *Psycho-Nutrition,* New York, NY: Grosset & Dunlap Publishing, 1976.

Fromm, Erich, *The Art of Loving,* New York, NY: Harper & Row Publishing, 1956.

Gendlin, Eugene T., *Focusing,* New York, NY: Everest House Publishers, 1978.

Goldberg, Herb, *The Hazards of Being Male,* New York, NY: The New American Library, 1976.

Goleman, Daniel, "Denial & Hope," *American Health,* December 1984, pp. 54-59.

Goulart, Frances Sheridan, *The Vegetarian Weightloss Cookbook,* New York, NY: Simon & Schuster, 1982.

Gygi, C., C. Saslow, C. B. Sengstake, and M. Whitman, "Self-confrontation and Weight Reduction: A Controlled Experiment," *Psychotherapy: Theory, Research and Practice,* 1973, pp. 10, 315-320.

Haas, Robert, *Eat To Win,* New York, NY: Rawson Associates, 1984.

Hamschck, Don E., "Psychodynamics of Normal and Neurotic Perfectionism," *Psychology,* 1978, pp. 27-33.

Harris, M. B., "Self-directed program for weight control — a pilot study," *Journal of Abnormal Psychology,* 1969.

Harris, M. B. and C. G. Bruner, "A comparison of a self-control and a contract procedure for weight control," *Behavior Research and Therapy,* 1971.

Hodgson, Ray and Peter Miller, *Self-Watching — Addictions, Habits, Compulsions: What to do About Them,* New York, NY: Facts On File Inc., 1982.

Jampolsky, Gerald G., *Love Is Letting Go Of Fear*, Millbrae, CA: Celestial Arts, 1979.

Jenkins, David C., "Psychosocial Modifers of Response to Stress," *Journal of Human Stress*, December 1979, 5:4, pp. 3-15.

Jourard, S., "Experimenter-subject Dialogue: A Paradigm for a Humanistic Science of Psychology In Beugental," J.F.T., *Challenges of Humanistic Psychology*, New York, NY: McGraw-Hill, 1967.

Katahn, Martin, "Obesity," *Encyclopedia of Clinical Assessment*, San Francisco, CA: Jossey-Bass Publishers, Henley Robert Woody, Editor, 1981, 1:319.

Kelly, A. H. and J. P. Curran, "Comparison of A Self-Control Approach To An Emotional Coping Approach To The Treatment of Obesity," *Journal Of Consulting and Clinical Psychology*, 1976, pp. 44, 683.

Kendall, Philip C. and Bemis M. Kelly, "Thought & Action In Psychotherapy: The Cognitive Behavioral Approaches," *The Clinical Psychology Handbook*, New York, NY: Pergaman Press, Michel and Belleck Hersen, Alan E. Kazdin, Editors, 1983, p. 565.

Kiester, Edwin Jr., "The Playing Fields of the Mind," *Psychology Today*, July 1984, pp. 18-24.

Kiester, Edwin Jr., "The Uses of Anger," *Psychology Today*, July 1984, p. 26.

Leon, G. and L. Roth, "Obesity: Psychological Causes, Correlations and Speculations," *Psychological Bulletin*, 1977, pp. 84, 117-139.

Leon, G. R. and K. Chamberlain, "Comparison of daily eating habits and emotional states of overweight persons successful or unsuccessful in maintaining a weight loss," *Journal of Consulting and Clinical Psychology*, 1973.

Leonard, George, "On Owning Our Power," *Association for Humanistic Psychology*, November 1975, pp. 178-180.

Leonard, George, *The Silent Pulse*, New York, NY: Bantam Books, 1978.

Lappe, Frances Moore, *Diet For A Small Planet*, New York, NY: Ballantine Books, 1976.

LeShan, Lawrence, *How To Meditate*, Boston, MA: Little, Brown and Co., 1974.

Lichtenberg, James W., "On Potential," *Journal of Conseling and Development*, October 1984, 63:101-102.

Linn, Robert, *The Last Chance Diet*, New York, NY: Bantam Books, 1977.

Locke, Steven E., and Mady Hornig-Rahan, *Mind and Immunity*, New York, NY: Institute for Advancement of Health, 1984.

Loring, Honey, *You're on — Teaching Assertiveness & Communication Skills*, Putney, VT: Stress Press, 1984.

MacLaine, Shirley, *Out On A Limb*, New York, NY: Bantam Books, 1984.

Mahoney, M. and K. Mahoney, *Permanent Weight Control: A Total Solution To The Dieter's Dilemma*, New York, NY: W. W. Norton, 1980.

Mandler, George, *Mind and Body*, New York, NY: W.W. Norton & Company, 1984.

Martin, Robert, "A Critical Review of The Concept of Stress in Psychosomatic Medicine," *Perspectives in Biology and Medicine*, Spring 1984, 27:3, pp. 443-464.

May, Rollo, *The Discovery of Being*, New York, NY: W. W. Norton, 1983.

McArthur, L. L., M. R. Soloman and R. H. Jaffe, "Weight Differences In Emotional Responsiveness to Proprioceptive and Pictorial Stimuli," *Journal of Personality and Social Psychology, 1980*, pp. 39, 308-319.

McCamy, John and James Presley, *Human Lifestyling*, New York, NY: Harper and Row Publishing, Inc., 1975.

McClelland, David C., "Power Is The Great Motivator," *Harvard Business Review*, March/April 1976, pp. 54, 100-111.

McClelland, David C., *Human Motivation*, Glenview, IL: Scott Foresman & Company, 1985.

McClelland, Floor, Erik and Richard J. Davidson and Saron Clifford, "Stressed Power Motivation," *Journal of Human Stress*, June 1980, pp. 11-19.

McClernan, James, "Are You An Emotional Eater," *Modern Bride*, October/November 1983, pp. 24, 26, 267, 269.

McClernan, James, "Falling For Food," *Shape*, February 1985, pp. 68-72.

McClernan, James, "Is Fear Keeping You Fat, *Shape*, May 1983, pp. 46, 47, 50, 86.

McClernan, James, "You Can Defeat The Mañana Syndrome," *Shape*, January 1985, pp. 78, 79-83.

McClernan, James and George L. Lawrence, "The Use of Existential and Behavioral Principles In A Comprehensive Treatment Program for Obesity," *Unpublished Paper,* Shick's Shadel Hospital Burien, Washington, D.C., March 1976, pp. 1-25.

McLaughlin, Maureen, A. Bonaguro and Daren Sussman, "An Exploration of Health Counseling & Goal Attainment Scaling In Health Education Programs," *Josh,* 1984, 54:10, pp. 403-405.

Meier, Robert M. and Susan Sheffler, "The Perils of Perfectionism," *Success,* September, 1984, pp. 24-27.

Nash, Joyce D. and Linda Ormiston Long, *Taking Charge Of Your Weight & Well Being,* Palo Alto, CA: Bull Publishing Co., 1978.

"Obesity — you can lose weight," *Life and Health National Health Journey,* 1st, 1: 1974.

Ogilvie, Bruce C. and Maynard A. Howe, "Beating Slumps at Their Own Game," *Psychology Today,* July 1984, pp. 28-32.

Olbrisch, Mary Ellen, "Evaluation of a Stress Management Program for High Utilizers of a Prepaid University Health Service," *Medical Care,* February 1981, XIX:2, pp. 153-159.

Ornish, Dean, *Stress Diet & Your Heart,* New York, NY: Holt, Rinehart and Winston, 1982.

Ornstein, Robert E., *The Psychology of Consciousness,* New York, NY: Penguin Books, 1972.

Peele, Stanton, "Change Without Pain," *American Health,* January/February 1985, pp. 36-39.

Peele, Stanton, *Love and Addiction,* New York, NY: Taplinger Publishing Co., 1975.

Pelletier, Kenneth R., *Mind As Healer-Mind As Slayer,* New York, NY: Delta Books, 1977.

Penick, S. B., R. Billion, S. Fox and A. J. Stunkard, "Behavior Modification in the Treatment of Obesity," *Psychosomatic Medicine,* 1971.

Polhemus, Ted, and Jonathan Benthall, Editors, *The Body As A Medium of Expression,* New York, NY: E. P. Dutton & Co., Inc., 1975.

Pritikin, N. and P. McGrady, *The Pritikin Program For Diet and Exercise,* New York, NY: Grosset & Dunlap, 1979.

Prokop, David, "A Diet For Life," *Runner's World,* December 1984, pp. 60-68, 90.

Rand, C. S. and A. J. Stunkard, "Obesity and Psychoanalysis," *American Journal of Psychiatry*, 1978, pp. 135, 547-551.

Rand, C. S., and A. J. Stunkard, "Psychotherapy For Obesity," *Psychology Today*, March 1984, 9:10-11, Ref: Am. Journal of Psychiatry, 140:9, New England Journal of Medicine, Vol. 309.

Resnick, H. and P. Balch, "The Effects of Anxiety and Response Cost Manipulations On The Eating Behaviors of Obese and Normal Weight Subjects," *Addictive Behaviors*, 1977, pp. 2, 219-225.

Rigden, Scott, *Take It Off!* — *The Weight Workbook*, Byron, IL: Lifestyle Communications, 1983.

Rorvik, David M., "How Your Diet Can Affect Your Mind," *McCall's*, April 1972, pp. 39-46.

Rossi, E. and S. Rossi, *Hypnotic Realities*, (Milton Erickson), New York, NY: Irvington Publishing, Inc., 1976.

Rubenstein, Carin, "Wellness Is All," *Health Survey Report, Psychology Today*, October 1982, pp. 28-37.

Rubin, Theodore Iszac, *Overcoming Indecisiveness*, New York, NY: Harper & Row, 1985.

Sachs, Michael L. and G. W. Buffone, Editors, *Running As Therapy*, Lincoln, NE: University of Nebraska Press, 1984.

Schachter, Stanley, and Robert J. Nivin, "Good News About Bad Habits," *Newsweek*, September 1982, p. 86.

Schutz, Wil, *Profound Simplicity*, New York, NY: Bantam Books, 1979.

Severin, Frank T., "What Humanistic Psychology Is About," *Association for Humanistic Psychology Journal*, January 1982, p. 92.

Shainess, Natalie, *Sweet Suffering* — *Woman As Victim*, Indianapolis, IN: The Bobs-Merrill Co., Inc., 1984.

Shapiro, Leona, Patricia Crawford and Ruth Huenemann, "A Time For Plumpness," *University of California Berkeley, Wellness Newsletter*, March 1985, p. 2.

Sheehan, George, *Running & Being*, New York, NY: Warner Books, 1978.

Siroka, Robert W., Ellen K. Siroka and Gilbert A. Schloss, *Sensitivity Training & Group Encounter*, New York, NY: Grosset & Dunlap, 1971.

Spino, Mike, *Beyond Jogging*, New York, NY: Berkley Publishing Corp., 1977.

Stuart, R. B., "A Three-dimensional Program for the Treatment of Obesity," *Behavior Research and Therapy,* 1971.

Stuart, R. B., "Behavioral Control for Overeating," *Behavior Research and Therapy,* 1967.

Stuart, R. and B. Davis, *Slim Chance In A Fat World: Behavioral Control of Obesity,* Champaign, IL: *Research,* 1978.

Stunkard, A. J., "The Success of Tops, A Self-help group," *Postgraduate Medicine,* 1972.

Stunkard, A. J. and Hume McLaren, "The Results of Treatment for Obesity: A Review of the Literature and Report of a Series," *Archives of Internal Medicine,* 1959.

Stunkard, A. J. and J. Reader, "The Management of Obesity," *New York Journal of Medicine,* 1958.

Travis, John, *Wellness Workbook,* Mill Valley, CA: Wellness Resource Center, 1977.

Tubesing, Nancy Loving, and Donald A. Tubesing, *Structured Exercises In Wellness Promotion, Vol. I,* Duluth, MN: Whole Person Press, 1983.

Walford, Roy L., *Maximum Lifespan,* New York, NY: Avon Books, 1983.

Watson, George, *Nutrition and Your Mind,* New York, NY: Bantam Books, 1972.

White, Boskind Marlene and William C. White Jr., *Bulimarexia,* New York, NY: W. W. Norton & Co., 1983.

Index

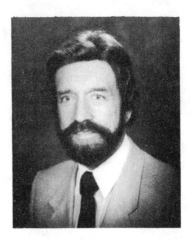

ABOUT THE AUTHOR

Dr. James McClernan is a leader in the human potential movement. He is a psychologist who has taught and counseled at several state universities and hospitals and who has consulted with business and industry. He is a former captain in the Bio-medical Corps of the US Air Force, and past president of two holistic health associations in Washington and Arizona. CHANGE YOUR MIND/CHANGE YOUR WEIGHT is based on his hospital research in Seattle, Washington and his many years of working with clients in private practice.

Dr. McClernan has published several articles in professional publications as well as popular women's and fitness magazines. He has made many successful radio and television appearances. He currently resides in Phoenix, Arizona, where he serves on the staff of John C. Lincoln Hospital in the Health Promotions Department, in addition to which he is Director of Programs and Development for the Human Dynamics Institute in Phoenix. Together with a medical doctor and an insurance firm, Dr. McClernan developed the W.I.S.E. Indicator©, a health risk assessment which is intended to aid in the reduction of health care costs. Research in psychoimmunology is Dr. McClernan's salient interest.